Mantras
Words of Power

MANTRAS
Words of Power

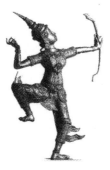

Swami Sivananda Radha

REVISED EDITION

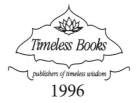

Timeless Books
publishers of timeless wisdom
1996

TIMELESS BOOKS
PO Box 3543
Spokane, WA 99220-3543
(509) 838-6652

In Canada: Timeless Books, Box 9, Kootenay Bay, B.C. V0B 1X0
        Phone: (604) 227-9224

In England: Timeless Books, 7 Roper Rd., Canterbury, Kent CT2 7EH
        Phone: (01227) 768813

Third printing
Printed in the United States of America

**Audio cassette tapes of Mantras are available from Timeless Books.
For information on classes in Mantras write Yasodhara Ashram, PO
Box 9, Kootenay Bay, B.C., Canada.**

Cover design by Laurel-Lea Shannon
Interior design by Deborah Pohorski
Photos for the revised edition by Joanne Pittman

Library of Congress Cataloging-in-Publication Data:
        Sivananda Radha, Swami, 1911-1995
                Mantras: Words of Power/Swami Sivananda Radha. --
                Rev. ed.
                        p.   cm.
                Includes bibliographical references and index.
                ISBN 0-931454-66-2 (paper) $14.95
                1. Mantra.   2. Yoga.   I. Title
        BL 1236.36.S58   1994
        294.5'37—dc20   93-46477
                                                            CIP

Published by

Timeless Books
publishers of timeless wisdom

Dedicated to Swami
Sivananda Saraswati of
Rishikesh India and all the
Gurus before him who have
prepared the Path.

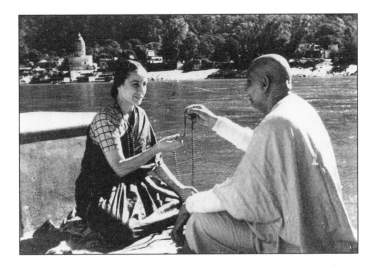

*Know that by prostration, by question and service,
the wise who have realised the Truth will instruct thee
in that knowledge.* FROM THE BHAGAVAD GITA

PHOTO: Swami Radha receiving her mala from Swami Sivananda on the day of
her Mantra initiation in India in 1956

Contents

	A WORD FROM THE AUTHOR	XV
	PREFACE	XXV
ONE	What is Mantra?	1
TWO	Mantra & Japa Yoga	9
THREE	Mantra Practice	15
FOUR	Worship: Cultivating the Imagination	29
FIVE	Benefits of Using a Mantra	37
SIX	How to Use the Mantra	49
SEVEN	Individual Mantras	63
EIGHT	Mantra & Healing	93
NINE	Mantra & Initiation	101
TEN	Experiences with mantra	111
ELEVEN	Mantra in Your Life	131
	APPENDIX	135
	SUGGESTED READING	159
	INDEX	165
	ABOUT THE AUTHOR	176

LIST OF ILLUSTRATIONS

The Archer, a Thai sculpture   COVER

Swami Radha receiving her mala from Swami Sivananda   P.VII

*Swami Nada Brahamananda giving Swami
    Radha a music lesson*   P.XVII

*Swami Venkatesananda playing the veena for
    Swami Sivananda*   P.XVII

*Swami Radha, Swami Venkatesananda, and Swami
    Nada Brahmananda playing on the banks of the Ganges*   P.XVIII

Gurudev Sivananda playing the harmonium   P.XXII

Swami Sivananda Saraswati seated on a tiger skin   P.XXIII

Swami Radha offering Namaste   P. 7

Bow and arrow (Likhita Japa)   P.12

Baby Krishna, the stealer of butter (Likhita Japa)   P.13

Radha and Krishna: humanity eternally seeking the Divine   P.24

Buddha   P.25

Krishna (Likhita Japa)   P.26

*The Temple of Divine Light Dedicated to All Religions at
    Yasodhara Ashram in British Columbia, Canada*   P.27

Lord Siva, with an offering of flowers   P.33

Black Madonna (needlepoint) P.34

Tara, an embroidery by the author P.35

Baby Krishna P.46

Krishna, the flute player P.47

White Tara (Likhita Japa) P.60

Radha and Krishna P.61

Tara, granter of boons P.73

Kuan Yin, goddess of compassion P.74

Krishna lures the devotee with His flute (batik) P.90

Nataraja Siva P.91

Kuan Yin P.91

Mary, Queen of Heaven P.99

An aspirant making an offering P.109

Siva dancing in a ring of fire P.127

Hanuman, loyal friend to Rama P.128

Tara (a gift from the Ganden Choeling Nunnery) P.129

Reclining Buddha P.129

ACKNOWLEDGEMENTS

The publication of this book and the previous edition are the result of many years preparation, involving the patience, time, and energy of a team of individuals who have both knowingly and unknowingly made their contributions.

My gratitude goes first to my great Guru, Swami Sivananda, to whom this book is dedicated, and to those who were my teachers at Sivananda Ashram in India: Swami Nada Brahmananda, my music guru, who instructed me in Mantra chanting; Swami Venkatesananda who, when I went through arduous training and despaired, would quietly play on his veena and lift my spirits by the power of the Mantra; Professor Shastri who gave me the theory and history of Mantras; and to Swami Saradananda who took some of the photographs.

There have been many others who have given encouragement and financial assistance. In the actual production of the book, the high quality of the editors and designers is evidence of their dedication to the Work. For their work on this revised edition in particular, I wish to thank Karin Lenman, Deborah Pohorski, Joanne Pittman, Norman MacKenzie, and Laurel-Lea Shannon.

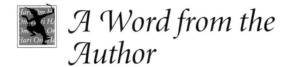# A Word from the Author

I knew nothing of Mantra before I went to India to meet Swami Sivananda Saraswati. As a child growing up in Germany I had many out-of-the-ordinary experiences and perceptions and, although I did not know enough to think of it that way, I used to sit in meditation—deep, deep in thought looking at one spot. My mother tried to discourage these strange ways and interest me in doing the things young girls usually do.

When I went to India in 1955 I heard about Mantras and the marvelous power they have, but I was Western and very skeptical. I asked my Guru what good repeating the same words over and over would do. He replied that I would have to practice chanting Mantra and find out. Through my practice of Mantra and keeping notes—I would record most of the times when I reached "impasses" as I called them, times when I just did not know why I was doing this practice—I recognized the rebellion of my mind.

It complained about carrying on something that seemed useless to it. But I continued—five hours a day, seven days a week, for seven weeks.

Swami Sivananda told me that I should intersperse the chanting with worship. When I said that I came from a Protestant religion and had no interest in ritual, he suggested something simple and beautiful, that I grow flowers of different colors and place them on an altar when I chanted. He said that I should always designate the same spot in my house as a holy place, and when I placed white flowers there, by the law of thought association, they would put me in touch with the spirit that is expressed in the symbol of Lord Siva. When I placed blue flowers on the altar, I would be put in touch with Lord Krishna, and roses or any colorful flower would bring me into touch with Divine Mother.

By this time Swami Sivananda had explained the male-female duality in the pantheon of the gods and goddesses of the Indian religions. To help me understand, he compared this to the family unit in the villages where one always knows the mother of a child, but not always the father. One can always recognize the power manifest— the female aspect, Divine Mother, or Sakti—but one cannot always recognize power unmanifest, the male, as symbolized by Lord Siva. I reflected on this and thought, "Yes, I can incorporate that into my thinking. When I grow white flowers for Siva I will remember that white has all colors, and Siva is energy, power. It is hard to think of energy, but the very fact that I know the symbol represents energy will help me. Swami Sivananda is not asking me to worship an image of Siva." I had the insight that the meditation on Lord Siva did not need to end with his image, that the image just became a focal point for my mind until I

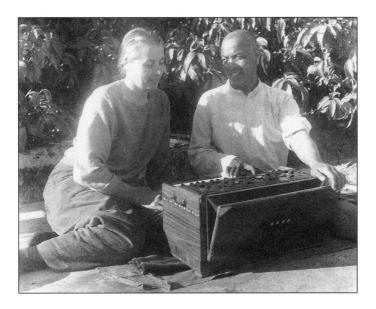

Swami Nada Brahamananda giving Swami Radha a music lesson

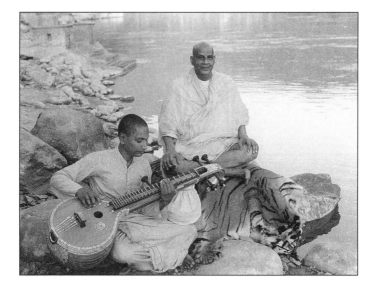

Swami Venkatesananda playing the veena for Swami Sivananda

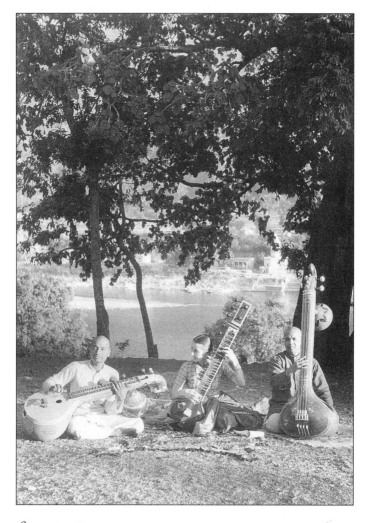

Swami Radha, Swami Venkatesananda, and Swami Nada Brahmananda playing on the banks of the Ganges

understood on a deeper level, intuitively, the principle of energy as such.

Back in Canada, I did not feel strong in my spiritual practice; my concentration was on a teeter-totter. The strangeness of these images helped me to focus, because although they were human figures I could not mistake them for any person I knew. In particular, the symbolic meaning of the bent position of Lord Krishna was helpful—"I am lenient with you, I am aware of your human failings. You keep forgetting your divine nature on account of the body, but I will remind you."

I thought in the same way about Divine Mother, and then I began to understand that a religion that has both the male and female aspects is bound to survive. I could see why Buddhists have the Mother of Compassion, and why Catholics have placed so much emphasis on Mary.

It was not easy, but I learned many things. As I had not had time to read books, what I did learn came to me from my own experience. I became aware of the impasses of the mind, the obstacles that the mind creates. I became aware of habit; habit had suggested to me that I would not be able to accomplish this chanting, that I would reach an impasse. If I had not made this suggestion to myself, or had not accepted the disparaging remark of someone I looked to as an authority, I might have had less difficulty.

I also had the problem of being sure that I had completed an accurate number of repetitions. When I chanted my Mantra, I used a box of matches and my mala with 108 beads. Every time I finished one mala I would throw one match on the floor. When I had finished ten malas I thought, "Well, I have done eighty extra Mantras. What shall I do with them?" I decided to make it 1100, simply to overcome the resistance of my mind. Slowly I got hold of myself.

The side effects of this were remarkable. My very depressive moods, in which I could see no purpose in life, all lifted. I had been given every material thing I wished for but did not find it worth living for that. Nor did I find it worthwhile to live for a marriage, when I saw all the problems of married life. But I felt there must be happiness somewhere since there were so many stories that we have descended from heaven. And then I wondered, "Is it possible for anyone to think of anything that has not existed at some time in the past or might exist at some time in the future?" The story of Icarus in Greek mythology came to my mind, the man who wished to fly. I thought that this may have been the beginning of the airplane. Maybe these things have to be imagined and desired in the mind to bring about the manifestation. It was the same principle Swami Sivananda had told me about—power unmanifest—so I asked, "What can I manifest? What will sound manifest? Do sounds manifest at all?"

I was probably very hard on myself. I would sometimes get up and walk around the prayer room to stop myself from falling asleep until I had finished my practice. When I went to China, I discovered that the monks there often walk as long as sixteen hours in spiritual practice, but I was only walking to keep myself awake until I had finished my Mantra repetitions.

I became aware of numerous things about the voice. For example, when someone pronounces my name, I know from the resonance of the voice if that person is friendly and likes me, or is really cool, reserved and distant, and only being socially polite. So many people are unaware of the messages they give, how even with a simple word they give themselves away. So I began to understand that there was something in the practice of chanting Mantras, after all.

Then some very beautiful things happened. I saw clouds of colors—lovely shades of blue. I thought of what blue meant—the blue Monday when people are depressed and not very active; the beautiful blue of the sky that makes everyone happy. Lord Krishna is presented as blue, and this shade of blue has become anchored in my mind as Krishna blue. The fleeting thought came to my mind that I must study symbolism. I noticed that after I had seen these beautiful shades of blue when chanting I was elated for a long time.

After some time I understood that I was becoming self-indulgent, and I said, "Oh, no, I am looking forward to something like spiritual movies. When will I ever stop looking for entertainment and comfort?" That is disastrous. Then one day I had an experience in which I maintained awareness. The sounds became like huge soap bubbles and they were spinning around; they had a kind of color and yet they didn't. Suddenly the desire surged up in me, "I wish I could sit on one and travel into space." At that very moment I saw myself move into space. That experience showed me that there is more than one way of leaving the body. I did not have the connection of a silver cord as I had heard of in others' experiences; there was nothing tugging at me. Then I began to wonder if my experiences were genuine since they were not like other people's, but I remembered my Guru saying, "Competition is not desirable. Although it is tolerated in business, it should not exist on the spiritual path," and I stopped making comparisons.

These experiences became a tremendous foundation and source of strength to help me carry on when my mind became restless, when it tried to revolt against this new discipline. My Guru, my great Guru, was a wonderful inspiration. I wanted to make real changes in myself and any pain and any effort were worth it.

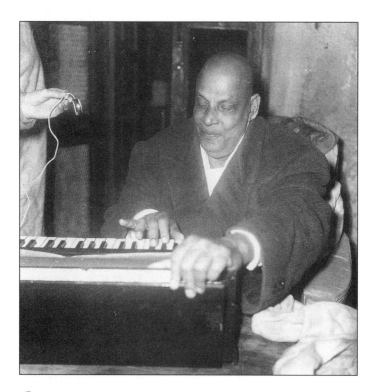

Gurudev Sivananda playing the harmonium

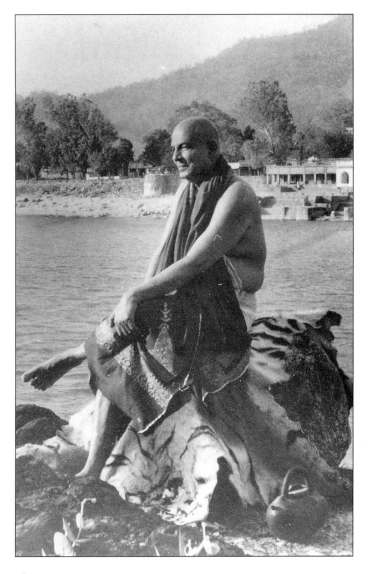

Swami Sivananda Saraswati seated on a tiger skin

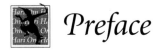 *Preface*

There is much that could be written on Mantra—there are, for example, many different kinds of Mantra—but this book is not intended to be a scholarly work on the subject. It is, rather, a practical guide to help people with their development in spiritual life through the practice of Mantra. However, it is helpful to know something about the place of Nada Yoga, the yoga of sound, in the philosophy of yoga, and in particular about that part of it known as Mantra Yoga.

The goal of all yoga is revelation, union with the Divine. Different paths of yoga have been followed in different ages, or "yugas" as they are sometimes referred to. In each yuga the goal of yoga is fulfilled in the way best suited to the individual in that particular age. Each yuga has had its yogis, teachers, or saints to show aspirants the way. These are holy people who have understood the emphasis of their particular time. In the Satya Yuga, for example (satya means purity), it was not necessary for the aspirants to do very much Hatha Yoga, or Bhakti or Jnana Yoga; the emphasis was on meditation. In the Treta Yuga sacrifice was recommended. This did not need to be the sacrifice of life; it might be the sacrifice of the desires of life, desires that are not really deep and that would have meant fulfillment only on the level of daily life. In the Dvapara Yuga all forms of worship were encouraged, prayers, conversations with God, worship in the highest form.

We are now said to live in the Kali Yuga, the Iron Age, the last of the four yugas, the evil age. Evil forces and immorality will prevail it is said, and this certainly seems to be so. At this time, Mantra Yoga, the chanting of the Lord's name, is supposed to be the best help for the development of the individual. There is a saying, *Kali Yuga Keval Namah Adhara,* which means, "In the Kali Yuga the holy name is the boat to cross the ocean of maya (illusion)."

Tradition says that the Mantras were given to us by the *rishis,* the great seers, holy ones and teachers who lived in times past. They, in turn, are said to have picked up the Mantras, or tuned into them, on the etheric level. The Mantras were created from the subtle vibrations of many millions of people who have cried out in their distress across the centuries. The Mantras are, so to speak, the essence of all those cries, but they are more than that; they are the answers to those cries.

Indian sages for hundreds of years have made a very detailed study of the effects of sound or, more correctly, of vibration. They are well aware of the power of sound in healing and in awakening the chakras (the centers of consciousness) in the Kundalini system.

Sound is vibration. Sounds and images have a very close relationship. In his book, *Japa Yoga,* Swami Sivananda gives several examples of singers who could produce images simply by singing a certain note or combination of notes. The creation of a particular sound may cause some material on that same rate of vibration to come together again. If the rate of vibration of the sound created is stronger and higher than that of an existing object, the object will break. With the correct sound, you can shatter glass. An Old Testament story tells of the sound of trumpets bringing down the walls of Jericho. The ear itself can be damaged by sound as we know from the unhappy stories of young people who suffer hearing loss because they listen to rock music that is played far too loudly.

A Mantra is sung to a melody, known as the *raga*. Raga (or ragini) is the Indian term for melody or key, but it includes much more than our idea of tune. Literally, raga means love or passion. It is a sound composition consisting of melodic movements that color one's heart.

The raga of a Mantra is primarily a monophonic one, a sequence of single sounds without harmony. In the teachings of Pythagorus it is pointed out that music, as it was understood in ancient Greece, is linked to arithmetic. This view has been expressed in more recent times in the writing of the late P. D. Ouspensky. The term "music of the spheres" belongs to the Greeks as well as to the Orient. The Greeks linked sound and music with astronomy. Aristotle in his *Poetica* states that language, rhythm, and sound together make up poetry. However, he points also to another element which has neither name nor form, and that is the ability of both the power of the word and the power of sound to influence human thought. Yogis say that this influence is more far-reaching than it is generally believed to be. Music is not only an orderly system or arrangement of sounds, but a power that can and does have an effect on the hearer. Confucius, like Aristotle, claimed that music will influence people and lead them to either right or wrong action. It is interesting to discover that the Greeks also made the point that the established melody must not be changed because such "lawlessness" leads to destruction.

Mantra Yoga is part of Nada Yoga, the yoga of sound, and is only one of about forty different approaches to yoga. Nada Yoga is a theory and understanding of sound, vibration, and music which has for centuries far exceeded any such understanding in the West. In this century, however, that understanding is being rediscovered by Western physicists as their work carries them beyond traditional ideas about the physical world.

Yogis have used the principles of Nada Yoga to bring themselves into harmony with the harmony of the Universe. In this book I have presented a practical way for beginning students to approach one part of Nada Yoga—Mantra Yoga—and to learn from personal experience of the great healing and unifying power of this practice.

MANTRAS: WORDS OF POWER

CHAPTER ONE

What is Mantra?

 A Mantra is a combination of sacred syllables which forms a nucleus of spiritual energy. This serves as a magnet to attract or a lens to focus spiritual vibrations. According to the Upanishads, the ancient scriptures of India, the original abode of the Mantra was the *Parma Akasha* or primeval ether, the eternal and immutable substratum of the universe, out of which, in the uttering of the primal sound *Vach,* the universe itself was created. (A similar account is found in the Gospel of St. John, "In the beginning was the Word. . . .") The Mantras existed within this ether and were directly perceived by the ancient rishis, or seers, who translated them into an audible pattern of words, rhythm, and melody.

Mantra is not prayer. Prayer consists of words of supplication chosen by the spiritual aspirant, whereas Mantra is a precise combination of words and sounds—

the embodiment of a particular form of consciousness or Sakti.

The root *man* in the word *Mantra* means in Sanskrit "to think;" *tra* comes from *trai,* meaning "to protect or free from the bondage of *samsara* or the phenomenal world." Therefore *Mantra* means "the thought that liberates and protects." But there are many levels of meaning in a Mantra which must be experienced to be truly understood. An intellectual explanation encompasses only a very small part of its meaning.

The chanting or recitation of Mantras activates and accelerates the creative spiritual force, promoting harmony in all parts of the human being. The devotee is gradually converted into a living center of spiritual vibration which is attuned to some other center of vibration vastly more powerful. This energy can be appropriated and directed for the benefit of the one who uses it and for that of others.

Every Mantra has six aspects: a *rishi* or seer, a *raga* or melody, the *Devata* or presiding deity, a *bija* or seed sound, the *Sakti* or power, and a *kilaka* or pillar.

The *rishis,* through their intuitive perception, opened themselves to the revelation of the Mantras and were able to recognize their own effectiveness as channels for the flow of grace, knowledge, and power from the Divine. These ancient seers understood that their powers were intended to be used in the service of others, as a guide to humankind.

The Mantras were transmitted from generation to generation, from Guru to disciple, and in this process the power of the Mantras was greatly increased. The repetition billions of times by countless devotees over the centuries has brought about a vast reservoir of power which augments the inherent spiritual potency of the Mantras.

The *raga* is comparable to a western melody line—a sound, or sequence of single sounds, without harmony. When chanting a Mantra it is extremely important not to change the raga and its key, because the rate of vibration on which the sound is based is an integral part of the Mantra. All Indian music is based on the understanding that there are two aspects to every sound: the audible expression, and the subtle sound-essence which carries the meaning and which arises from the eternal Spirit. This essence is called *Shabda* or *Vach*. When the spoken word is perfectly sounded within and without, contact is made with this power which manifests as an image.

There is a certain power in a word even on a human level—one's own name has a special significance, and the way in which it is pronounced can convey numerous messages. Different tones cause different vibrations affecting the bodily, as well as the emotional, response. The practice of Mantra Yoga for a long period of time makes one aware of sounds actually creating images, and of certain images having an inherent sound.

In his book, *Japa Yoga,* Swami Sivananda says that sounds are vibration which give rise to definite forms. The repeated chanting of the name of the Lord gradually builds up the form or special manifestation of the deity worshipped (the Devata) and acts as a focus to concentrate this influence, which then penetrates and becomes the center of consciousness of the worshipper.

The *Devata* is the presiding deity of the Mantra, the informing power, a very personal aspect of God. It is the wisdom that comes from a higher source and is like a single beam of sunlight, one beam that is singled out and given a name so that the disciple can develop a personal relationship with and worship an aspect of God that he or she can understand. Or it may be likened to one facet of a diamond representing Cosmic Intelligence. A diamond with many facets will reflect many rays of Light at the same time, but one particular ray will especially appeal to the individual as he or she begins travelling the spiritual path. In the beginning, God is too awesome for the human mind to grasp and only later can divine energy be perceived in its pure form, so the human mind needs to establish a link with a personal aspect such as Krishna or Siva in the Indian religions, or Jesus or Mary in Christianity. Adults who are still spiritual children need to have a personal concept of God until they can see the divine energy in its pure form.

The Mantras, *Om Krishna Guru* and *Hari Om,* and the *Krishna Invocation,* are associated with Krishna; *Om Namah Sivaya,* with Siva; and *Om Tara,* with Divine Mother. (See Chapter Seven for details of each Mantra.) If you think of the millions of people in India over the centuries who have chanted the name of Krishna or Siva, or all the Christians over the years who have repeated the name of Jesus, you can see that this constant repetition would create a tremendous reserve of power. The power of their achievement is present in the combined energy of the Mantra. The truly devout person who chants the name of a particular aspect of the Divine will eventually tap into that power of the Devata.

One drop of water can accomplish very little, but hundreds of millions of drops can cut through rock or, indeed, change the face of the earth.

Each Mantra has a *bija* or seed. This is the essence of the Mantra and it gives the Mantra its special power—its self-generating power. Just as within a seed is hidden a tree, so the energy in the Mantra is the seed from which will grow a beautiful spiritual being. If you were to chant quite regularly now, abandon the practice, and then perhaps twenty years from now suddenly find yourself in some crisis, the Mantra might come automatically to your lips and you would continue to repeat it as if you had never ceased. This is an example of its self-generating power.

If you think of Shabda, the primal sound, the nuclear sound Om, from which all things are created, and bija the seed and self-generating power of the Mantra, you will see that through constant and correct chanting of a Mantra, you will be helped to release greater energy within your physical, mental, emotional, and spiritual bodies. With this increase of energy you will also be helped to get in touch with the Divine within you, your true Self, your Higher Self.

The *kilaka,* or pillar, is at first the driving force, the persistence and will-power that the disciple needs to pursue the Mantra. But when the power of the Mantra begins to take on a self-generating "flywheel motion," the kilaka becomes a very fine thread joining the disciple to the Mantra, to the power of the Mantra, to the Guru, and to the deity, until all become one.[1]

The power, the consciousness within the Mantra, is *Sakti,* Divine Mother, the Goddess of the Spoken Word. The male aspect of God is energy in a state of equilibrium; the female aspect is dynamic energy which manifests as creation. There is only one energy in all created things. In the Mantra that energy is present in pure form. The potency of the Mantra is released through repetition until

---

1   See Chapter Eleven for a description of an experience of the kilaka.

the individual finally comes to his or her Devata and a spiritual experience may take place.[2]

By constant recollection or thinking of the Mantra one is protected from the impact of *maya*, the illusory world. Through repetition of these words of power, the goal of Mantra Yoga is achieved—that is (as with all yogas) unity of individual consciousness with Cosmic Consciousness.

Mantra is the song of a star ...
and it will transport you to that star.

2　All consciousness is energy, a vortex of energy. It may be compared to the funnel of a tornado. This funnel does not actually exist; it appears because the currents of air pick up dust. When the tornado is over, the energy goes somewhere else and manifests in the same way or in a different way. Consciousness may be compared to that energy—it is indestructible. To give an example of how energy and image are associated, several years ago newspapers reported that the call letters and test pattern of a television station in the United States were picked up in the studio of a station in England. What was really curious was not that this signal had been picked up, but that that particular test pattern had not been used for five years. The energy manifested in it had drifted about in space all that time at the rate of 186,000 miles per second and then, apparently by chance, had come back to the planet earth.

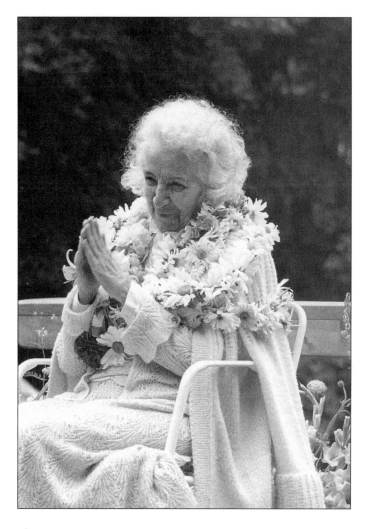

Swami Radha offering Namaste

CHAPTER TWO

Mantra & Japa

 Mantra Yoga is one of the manifold yogas, of which there are about forty, all inter-woven like threads of a cloth. The four principal ones are: Bhakti Yoga, the yoga of love and devotion; Karma Yoga, the yoga of action; Jnana Yoga, the yoga of knowledge and wisdom; and Raja Yoga, the "kingly yoga," a combination of several yogas based on the Yoga Sutras of Patanjali. One type of spiritual practice is sufficient to attain God-Realization, but since there is an interaction of the body forces, the yogas cannot be completely separated. Also because of physical problems, such as restlessness and poor blood circulation, it is recommended that several different yogas be included in a balanced practice.

The chanting of a Mantra is called Mantra Yoga. All other forms of repeating the Mantra are called *Japa Yoga*.

When the Mantra is spoken aloud, it is known as *Vaikhari Japa;* when whispered or hummed it is *Upamsu Japa;* when the repetition is mental it is called *Manasika Japa;* written Mantra is called *Likhita Japa.*

The use of Mantra in any of these forms is effective in securing single-pointedness of mind. The most subtle, Manasika Japa, although it is very powerful, may be difficult for those who are just beginning a Mantra practice. Alternating it with vocal repetition helps to keep the mind from wandering. Likhita can be done in any script, in any language, but should be consistent for the chosen length of time. This repetitive writing brings peace, poise, and strength within, and may also be used to alternate with the other forms of Japa.

Chanting a Mantra with devotion and concentration attunes the individual through divine melody and has a harmonious influence over the whole body and mind. It is important to use the correct raga (melody) always, since precise rules govern the interrelation and sequences of sound. Each raga, which is a particular combination of sound, is claimed to reflect the laws of the universe and to be in perfect harmony with the universe at the time it is sounded. Since sound results from the union of the breath and intellect of a human being, the one who chants will be brought to harmony also.

Chanting produces a series of psychological and spiritual effects. The concentration brings a deep sense of peace and joy, as often arises with other forms of meditation. The Mantra serves the same function as the *koan* in Zen or the mandala of Tibetan Buddhism: it functions as a device for focusing the ordinarily dispersed powers of the mind to a sharp point that is capable of penetrating through the sifting sands of thoughts to the deeper layers of mind beneath.

Through constant repetition of the Mantra one becomes like a magnet attracting the spiritual power of the Mantra to oneself and becoming aware of the Self. This repetition gradually awakens the higher faculties in a person and raises the consciousness toward the level of the mantric resonance. According to Vedic teaching, "A Mantra has the power of releasing the Cosmic and Supra-cosmic Consciousness," and it bestows freedom, ultimate illumination, and immortality.

Not only the singer benefits, but also those who listen and attune themselves to the spirit of the singing. This serves not only as an aid to meditation but is, in fact, a form of meditation in itself.

When a Mantra has been received from a Guru, the power of that Mantra increases after the initiation. In the Guru-disciple relationship, both are under an obligation throughout their lives to chant the Mantra which has been given to the disciple. It constitutes a permanent spiritual link between them. As the initiate practices, the Mantra becomes a self-generating force, uniting the individual with the power of the Mantra. Through his or her own efforts the disciple is drawn toward the chain of Gurus who have found Self-Realization through the use of the Mantra. In due time, the disciple must become a link in that chain.

By reciting the Mantra you carry its force and power, and this will be a blessing for all those you meet. At times the mantric power may take over so that it will not even be necessary to speak. As a person, as a mind, you do not need to get involved. This is a much more valuable communication which can take place on the soul level.

The practice of this form of yoga is as effective today as in former times, and is still taught and practiced by the Gurus and spiritual teachers of India. In fact, it is said that

Mantra Shastra[1] is the easiest means by which the aspirant may reach Self-Realization in the present era. Mantras are used at every significant step of religious life in the Indian spiritual tradition.

Mantra is an accumulation of power that is activated by the one who practices it, thereby drawing this power to oneself and merging in it through surrender. Through the use of Mantra, one becomes conscious of the self, beginning with a small "s." Expanding awareness will eventually lead one to become aware of the Self with a capital "S." This results eventually in achieving unity of the lower self and the Higher Self. Mantra leads the Spirit, lost in trivialities and worldly pursuits, back to pure Essence.

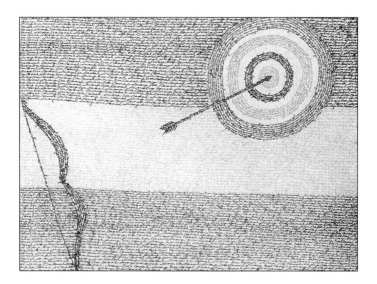

Bow and Arrow (Likhita Japa)

---

1   Mantra practice in accordance with the *Shastra* (scriptures).

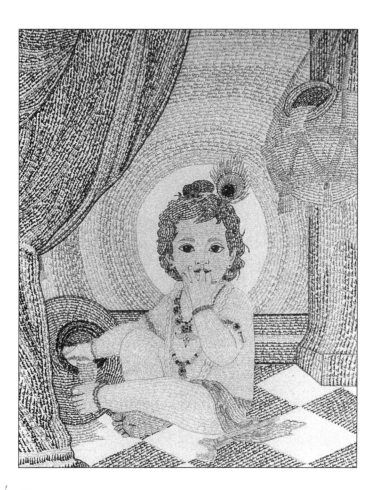

Baby Krishna, the stealer of butter (Likhita Japa)

CHAPTER THREE

Mantra Practice

 When you begin a Mantra practice you need to clarify to yourself what you want to achieve. What are your ideals? You can rightfully pin your hopes on the Mantra to help bring these ideals into manifestation in your life in the purest form possible. But to what extent and how soon this will come to pass depends on you. Obviously, the more you put into it the more you will achieve. The pearl exacts its price.

While you chant, observe the mind. You may be shocked at how easily the mind can be side-tracked and how quickly you get bored. You may even begin to doubt your sincerity in desiring God or desiring to become single-pointed, as you watch the mind finding dozens of excuses to stop chanting. Perhaps you will tell yourself that doing a charitable act would be a more worthwhile way to spend the time. But you are missing the point when you start thinking this way. You will be of far more help to others when you have gained some spiritual power.

The choice of Mantra is extremely important because the greatest success lies with the Mantra to which you can best surrender. There is a specific Mantra for each person—the *Ishta Mantra.* This does not mean that no two people will have the same Mantra. However, according to the principles of Nada Yoga, the yoga of sound, there is a particular sound, a particular vibration, to which your body will best respond. The Mantra that is designated for you corresponds to your spiritual nature.

There are many ways in which a Mantra may be chosen. You can chant a Mantra to which you simply feel drawn and naturally attracted. If you are fortunate enough to find a true Guru, your Guru may choose the Mantra to which you are best suited. You may ask your Guru for a certain Mantra, or it may be given to you by the Guru in a moment of inspiration. Or it may come to you in a dream.

Having chosen or been given your Mantra, stay with it until you have had some experience of its power. Resist the temptation to change to another one, thinking perhaps you made the wrong choice, or because you are bored, or because the high notes are too difficult for you to reach. Begin with one Mantra and lay a good foundation. Only at a much later stage of your development can you use two or three Mantras.

In the practice of Japa Yoga, a *mala* is used to assist in counting the repetitions of the name of a divine aspect such as Siva or Divine Mother. A mala is a string of 108 beads, usually made of sandalwood, tulsi, or rudraksha seeds. The number *108* is a holy number. *1* means one line, symbolizing God, the Supreme Energy, the power from which all other lines, circles, or movements come.

O is completeness, a circle representing God's creation as complete and perfect. 8, as the sign of eternity, brings in the time element, for creation goes on eternally. Time can be stretched or compressed. This understanding comes only through practice.

For the busy Western person especially, the practice of the mala has therapeutic value because of its effects of concentrating the mind, directing the emotions, and focusing the body, all of which lead to the spiritual realm.

The mind is constantly moving, using energy unproductively by creating mental background noises which are mainly concerned with past or future events. Life is an endless chain of cause and effect. The beads of the mala are also an endless chain and with each bead the endless thoughts are given a specified, significant meaning relating to the particular Mantra. There is a special bead called Mount Meru where the mala is tied together. When the fingers reach Mount Meru, the mala should be turned and the movement continued the other way. This bead symbolizes God-Realization and each time you reach it you have a reminder that you do not have to continue the chain of cause and effect. Another reminder is given in holding the mala at heart level, signifying the devotional aspect of this practice, the attempt to transcend the lower levels of being.

The use of a mala gives the body some activity and thereby releases nervous energy or restlessness. As the Mantra is repeated with each bead, the beads are moved between the third (ring) finger and the thumb, never the first (index) finger and thumb. Through use the beads take on some of the energy of the user and they become spiritualized. If the mala is made from the tulsi tree, it will be a little rough at first, but the beads will be made smooth by the practice. The mala should be worn around the neck with Mount Meru in front. Wearing the mala reminds you of your purpose in life, to realize God, the Self, because you feel it when you move in all your daily activities. Place it under your pillow or on your altar at night.

To get the greatest benefit from your Mantra practice, set a definite period of time aside each day and make a written commitment to yourself to continue the practice for a period of time long enough that you can feel its effects. Three months is a good beginning. Begin small and build up—this develops enthusiasm and perseverance to handle greater things. Do not be over-ambitious, letting the ego convince you that you will be able to sustain a long period of chanting immediately. Handle your spiritual growth with at least as much care as you would a little seedling, which needs the greatest care and attention. The recommended time for Mantra practice is four o'clock in the morning because at that hour there are few troubling vibrations in the air. However, this may be difficult unless you are living in an ashram or by yourself. When you set your time for practice, remember that you should not chant for at least an hour and a half after meals. As you become accustomed to the idea, increase the time of practice. You will become very conscious of time, how you spend it and how, perhaps, you waste it. Make a practice of writing down everything that you do in a day. See where you waste time and learn to be efficient so that you can find the time you want for spiritual practice.

Before beginning to chant take a bath, or at least wash your hands, face, and feet. As you wash, think that the impurities of your mind are being washed away. Put on fresh clothes and think that your soul is being clothed with a new garment of a divine nature. These thoughts will help to uplift you. Put into your mind a clear, commanding thought that your full attention will be given to chanting for a specific period of time. Free the mind of all other things by reviewing any worries or duties, firmly promising yourself that you will deal with them when your period of chanting is over but stating that they are not to intrude on the time you have set aside to be holy.

Choose a quiet spot where you will not be disturbed and use it each time, facing north or east. Sit in a comfortable chair or on the floor with a cushion. If a cushion is used for support of the back, be sure that it is placed below the waist to straighten the spine, not to fill in the curve at the waist. There is a subtle power in the thought of straightening the spine, suggesting straightforwardness, thinking straight, moving with uprightness and strength.

Place a pure wool blanket or a pure silk cloth to sit upon at the place you have chosen to do your practice. A deerskin or tiger skin are traditionally used for this purpose, to conserve energy and keep out the vibrations of the earth. We want to create a very different magnetism that will release us from the magnetism of the earth, from our needs and instincts, that will carry us to great heights of consciousness and awareness. Use also a shawl of natural fibre to cover the body as this will fulfill the same function and help to retain the spiritual vibrations you generate.

Sit cross-legged on the floor with the left leg over the right, or in one of the traditional yogic asanas such as *siddhasana* (the perfect pose), *padmasana* (the lotus), *virasana* (kneeling pose), or *sukhasana* (easy pose); or in a chair with your back straight. The spine must be straight so that the pranic current which is created or stimulated through the chanting can flow freely. A crooked spine is like a broken wire; sometimes the connection is made and sometimes it is not. From the yogic point of view this pranic circuit of the body should be closed by crossing the ankles to maintain the beneficial effects of the Mantra. Rest the hands in your lap, with the palms up, thus suggesting surrender and receptivity to divine insights.

Before beginning to chant make sure that the large muscles of your body are relaxed. Relax the neck and shoulders, as well, and also the muscles of the tongue, jaw, forehead, and eyes. Focus the eyes gently on the space between your eyebrows.

As you chant, pull the abdominal muscles in, thus forcing the air out of the lungs. As the air comes in, let the chest widen by itself, not by lifting the shoulders. Use all the breath, all your energy. Put yourself completely into your chanting. It is important to breathe through your nose. The right kind of deep breathing will naturally begin to take place when you chant; there is no danger, as there is with some breathing exercises. Watch your breath and keep expelling it evenly.

Learn to sit motionlessly for increased periods of time. Check the position of the body at the end of that time to be sure that your head, shoulders, and back are straight, but relaxed, with the vertebrae one on top of the other.

At the beginning and end of your practice, offer a prayer of thanksgiving to those who have chanted the Mantra. In this way you attract those who have found God-Realization by the use of the Mantra. If you say, "Help, help, please come and help me," they will come to support you. By accepting that this is possible, you help yourself to have the experience. Do not let your intellect decide what can or cannot be. Hold judgment suspended and see what happens.

The melody of the Mantra must never be changed. The combination of sounds is based on the perception of the rishis who translated the etheric vibrations into those particular combinations for the purpose of creating a magnetic effect in the human being. If you have difficulty in reaching the high notes, you must not change the key. The voice will adjust. Not being able to reach the high notes should be seen symbolically. Do not let the ego get in the way and discourage you from continuing. The voice needs training, and with time, patience, and practice it will rise to the higher notes. You will find your voice becoming clearer, smoother, and able to reach notes you never thought you would be able to sing. That is one of the little miracles along the way. Just as the voice needs training, the mind and consciousness also need to be trained with the same diligence to reach heights you never dreamed of.

Really put yourself into the chanting. If you allow it to become mechanical, or if you let yourself think it is monotonous, or if you let your interest drop, it will take a longer time to be effective. As with learning a language, the more you give yourself to it, the faster you will become fluent. When you study and practice Mantra you will learn the language of the Divine.

After your Mantra practice remain quiet and receptive, surrendering your will to the Divine. Allow the still, small voice to speak. Come out of your practice gently and slowly. Don't get up and rush into something new. Try to keep the sensitivity, peace, and quiet for as long as possible. Time is needed following spiritual practice for the effects to be absorbed. Take time also to reflect and write down your thoughts.

To summarize: First, set the length of time you will chant. Then, with a shawl around your shoulders, sit erect, relaxed, in a quiet place, on a piece of cloth of natural fi-bre, left leg crossed over right, hands in lap, palms up. Deal with objections and obstacles before you start to chant, offer a prayer of thanksgiving, then give yourself a clear commanding thought of what you are about to do. Focus attention on the space between the eyebrows. Begin to chant, drawing in the abdominal muscles to expel the air; as you breathe in, feel the chest widening. Put yourself into the chanting. Work at keeping the mind interested and concentrated. Stick to the length of time you have set to chant. Offer your prayer of thanksgiving again when you have finished chanting. Remain quiet and receptive for a period of time after chanting. Afterwards write down observations that come easily to mind. As time goes on you will find it revealing to read them over.

At times during your Mantra practice, you may get in touch with emotions you did not know you had. Tears may arise that may have been held back since childhood. These tears are nothing to be ashamed of. They may be tears of self-pity, or of regret at having wasted so many years. Sometimes they are a rejuvenating force that can refresh by washing away an accumulation of sadness. Swami Sivananda suggested that people collect their tears symbolically and wash the feet of Divine Mother with them. But do not indulge yourself in your tears. They represent a small progress, not a great one.

Sometimes people faint during chanting. This may occur in people with poor blood circulation after long periods of chanting. This will not have any after effect. Fainting may also occur, particularly in prolonged group chanting, because the atomic structure of the brain has to be changed to adjust to the new vibration to which it is being exposed. This is a genuine response to the power of the Mantra, and it will manifest as a noticeable change in the personality of the individual. There will be a tendency to rethink many concepts, and new ideals will be established. There will be a growing desire to break free from limitations, and a conscious striving to be on the spiritual path.

The student must learn how to control this energy when it arises. The method for doing so is very simple. It is necessary only to feel the feet placed firmly on the floor and to remind oneself that one is here, now, in the physical world. Human beings are the bridge between two worlds, the world of the physical, material body, and the unseen world created by the mind, which can manifest something through our belief in it.

Another technique to help control the sudden rush of this newly experienced energy is to visualize a beautiful golden lotus at the base of the spine. Then gently but firmly place the Light within the spine back into that lotus where it belongs, and close the petals securely around the Light. Again, remind yourself by an act of will to be here, now. It is very important not to indulge emotions, not to seek experience, not to try to bring on a similar experience by chanting very quickly or experimenting with a breathing technique. If you give in to this temptation, you will soon experience doubt, and begin wondering whether any experience is really a manifestation of the Divine or just an artificial production of your own imagination. Secondly, you will be caught up in the desire for experience, for sensation, and will not look beyond to see the true Light.

At a later date in your spiritual practice you may be faced with the temptation of *siddhis,* the powers of extrasensory perception. These powers may be used for good purposes, but too often they are only a temptation to the ego. If you give in to this temptation you may fall even further from your spiritual goal than you were before you started the practice of chanting Mantra.

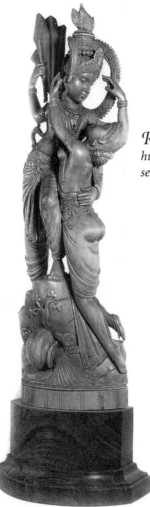

Radha and Krishna: humanity eternally seeking the Divine

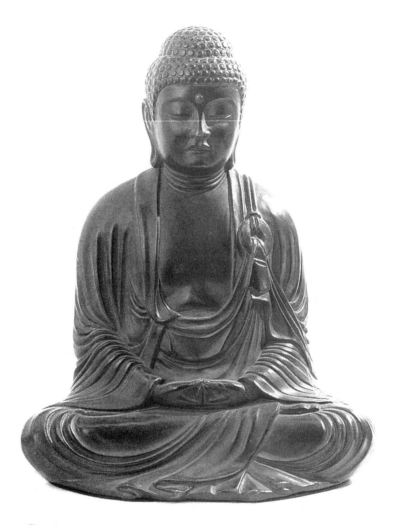

Buddha

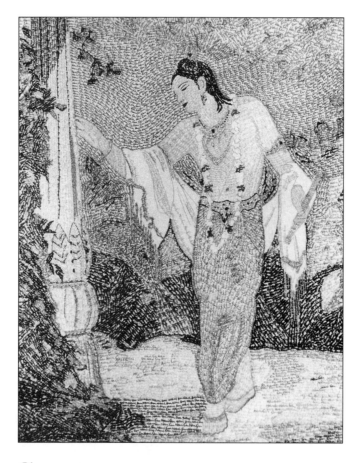

*K*rishna *(Likhita Japa)*

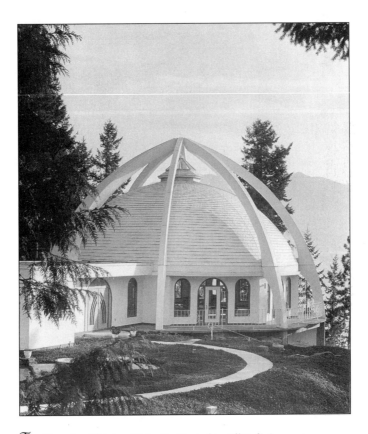

The Temple of Divine Light Dedicated to All Religions, at Yasodhara Ashram in British Columbia, Canada

CHAPTER FOUR

Worship: Cultivating the Imagination

 The mind needs a concrete image to keep it single-pointed during Mantra practice. In Bhakti Yoga, the yoga of love and devotion, the devotee concentrates on the picture of the deity connected with the Mantra. This deity, the *Ishta Devata*, creates a great longing in the devotee. There is a link of love and mercy, an extended help from the power of the deity, which the picture represents. This happens because of the complete surrender of the body, of the mind, and of the ego at the feet of the deity. The image stands for the Most High, everything that is holy, perfect, beautiful to the mind of the devotee, and there is a response of those qualities within the individual.

There is great wisdom in entering into a personal relationship with a particular aspect of the Divine. We can understand and see God only as an image we create in our mind, and we begin by creating God in our own image. You can paint an image, take one from a book, or you can use a picture of your spiritual teacher. This can be most helpful, since you already know what he or she looks like. You bring to life any image of the Divine that you charge with the power of your mind, your prayer, and your love. In this way you cultivate your imagination while practicing the Mantra.

These images of worship can also be invoked in the mind's eye, thus increasing the power of positive imagination. Desire is born out of imagination. In worship we put God into our mind so the Divine becomes part of our desire, and we raise the scheming for the fulfillment of desire to a higher level.

The eyes may be kept closed, focused on the space between the eyebrows. If the mind cannot be stilled when you are chanting, open your eyes and chant straight to heaven, invoking the name of God with a deep feeling of expectancy that Someone is really listening. Use the power of your imagination and, looking into the sky, imagine an enormous ear. Sing into this ear and see what happens. Or take an image of God and establish it firmly in your mind. Then try to reproduce it in the sky and feel a deep longing to be near God. Imagine Christ on the cross, or in a fishing boat calming the storm; or imagine Krishna, with his beautiful Indian jewelry, his peacock feather, his flute, his ankle-bells, and his blue skin which shows that he is God and not another human being, that he stands for the divine principle.

As a method of pacifying the rebellious mind and overcoming the temptation to be side-tracked, you can intersperse the recitation of Mantra with brief periods of worship, such as choosing and arranging flowers, making garlands, or caring for an altar, thus bringing into your consciousness that aspect of the Divine. First, designate and keep some spot in your home as a holy place in which to chant Mantra and offer worship. Then choose a ritual which suits you. Such rituals can help to focus the mind.

In the beginning, many people feel they need protection and the Siva Mantra may be the answer to that first impulse. To include worship of Lord Siva in your practice, it is sufficient to utter his name while dropping clear water over a stone representing him. Siva is the aspect of the Divine that the rishis recognized as the originator, the Sakta, the Lord of Kundalini and Hatha Yoga, which are very active practices calling for demanding discipline. But for those who do not have that ability, calling on Siva's name while pouring a little water over a Siva stone is adequate.

If your chosen deity is Lord Siva in the aspect of destroyer of all obstacles, you can grow white flowers and place them on an altar for him. By the law of thought association the white flowers will put you in touch with the snowy peaks of the Himalayas, the abode of Lord Siva. If you chant *Hari Om,* invoking the aspect of the Lord as Vishnu, the preserving one, you can use blue flowers. Roses or other colorful flowers may be used as an offering to Divine Mother when you use *Ave Maria* or *Om Tara* as your Mantra.

Place a flower, real or imagined, before an image of Christ, the Virgin Mother, Siva, Buddha, or whomever you wish. Then say, "God, here is a flower. I have not made the flower. I have no power to create a flower. I have really nothing, not a single thing I can call my own. But I take this little part of your creation and I give it back to you, charged with my love, my emotion, and my devotion. Please accept my offering." This gesture will help you to realize that only after you have done the preliminary work with your imagination can you recognize God in the flower or see the Divine Light in it.

You may put flowers on your altar, burn a candle, and say, "God, I wish you to accept the flowers as a symbol of my devotion; may the candle be a symbol of my false desires, and may they be burned in the Light of Wisdom as this candle burns before my eyes."

Put a little vessel of water on the altar and leave it there for three months without renewing the water. Every day drink just one sip and wonder as you experience that the water stays fresh as you raise the vibrations of your mind because of your chanting and prayers. Let each sip of water be symbolic of the Mantras and prayers that will wash away the debris of the mind. You may find that the water will remain fresh without being covered throughout the whole time of your spiritual practice. Do not be ashamed to perform such acts of worship. You have a right to expect a great deal, but you have to open the doors for something to happen.

Ritual should help the individual experience gratitude for knowledge of what any personalized aspect of the impersonal power truly represents. Worship of some aspects of the Divine may be more elaborate, but it is not necessary to make ritual complicated, as this may only burden the worshipper with details to the exclusion of the finer feelings.[1]

You may also embroider the picture of the Devata of

---

1 The subtlety of the psychology of these procedures, concepts, and attitudes may be more easily understood, however, if we remember that at the time of the development of such rituals, mechanical clocks did not exist, so the inner clock in human beings had to be developed. The practice or ritual alone, when done with precision, could lead the devotee to

your Mantra. While making each stitch, ask yourself questions such as, "Why is the skin this color? Why is the hand held in this position? What does this piece of jewelry symbolize?"

After some time is spent in cultivating the imagination through a variety of forms of worship, the mind may achieve a level of concentration in which it will willingly resort to more subtle images of the Divine, such as breath or Light.

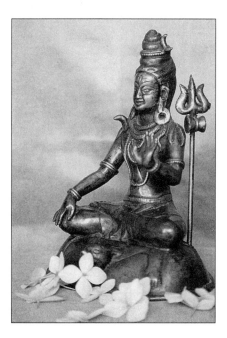

Lord Siva, with an offering of flowers

---

remarkable understanding. The early yogis realized that this was not the only way in which the mind could be trained, that in fact its powers could be vastly expanded. The desire to make oneself accessible to those powers, using the methods developed, can bring about an experience of greater Reality.

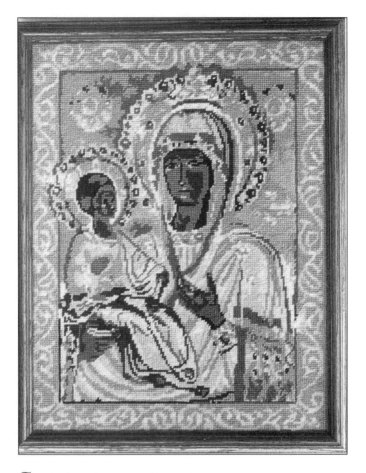

The Black Madonna (needlepoint)

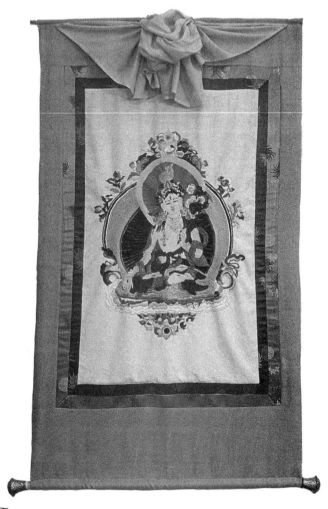

Tara, an embroidery by the author

CHAPTER FIVE

The Benefits
of Using Mantra

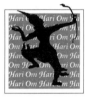 The repetition of a Mantra is a means of improving the powers of concentration. There are Indian spiritual masters who maintain that the meaning and the content of the Mantra do not necessarily have to be understood by the aspirant in order to bring about the desired effect, that the practice of Mantra alone is sufficient to achieve the spiritual awakening which is its purpose. Certainly, the use of the Mantra purifies the subconscious and even if it is repeated mechanically some purification will take place. However, each Mantra is devotional by nature and has the Divine as its form and essence. With concentration on the meaning, the attainment of the ultimate goal is surer and quicker.

The benefits of Mantra practice depend on you as an individual, on where you started off, where you stand now, what your past lives have been, and the intensity and degree of longing in your desire. When you chant a Mantra your whole being changes for the better. Build up the habit of repeating the Mantra at all times. The work you do will become easier and more joyful because the Mantra is continuously in the back of your mind.

One of the results that comes quickly with the practice of Mantra is control of the breath which is the means by which we can develop the ability to control the emotions. In chanting we can give all our emotions to the Mantra, to the deity of the Mantra, and ask that deity to help us gain control. In this way we find a safe release for negative feelings. Rather than throwing them on someone else, we offer them back to their source. Continued chanting will lead to greater awareness and the replacing of negative feelings with positive affirmations.

Mantra practice stills turbulent emotions and thereby stills the turbulent mind. In yogic terms there is a difference between emotions and feelings, since a purified emotion becomes a true feeling. Mantra Yoga gives us an opportunity to know the emotions, what they are, where they come from, and what their proper place is in our lives. Through Mantra Yoga we can learn to deal with the emotions properly, to control and refine them, and to encourage the harmonious development of all aspects of the human potential.

As the Mantra is put into the subconscious, the mind is purified to an extent of which we would be incapable without this aid. Slowly the ego is overpowered by the Higher Self. It is like pouring milk into a cup of black coffee until, little by little, the coffee is replaced by pure milk. Because it purifies the mind, the Mantra is also a great protection from fear.

When emotions are purified they develop into love, which is an important step in the awakening of further levels of consciousness, and the influence of the Mantra becomes very subtle. Feelings which have been purified bring us into the presence of the Divine and from the Divine we feel a sense of protection. The Mantra is like a shield against all that is negative and disturbing.

Although you may have experienced fears, worries, loneliness, and only limited encounters with love and joy, do not despair. Even if your feelings are easily hurt, in that over-sensitivity you have a wonderful, if as yet undeveloped, tool. As these negative emotions evolve into more refined feelings, you will find that your concepts of love and joy also change, and that such sensitivity is exactly what is needed to enter new dimensions of understanding on the path to Self-Realization.

The voice can become an instrument for expressing and controlling the emotions. Even if you cannot reach the high notes in the beginning, you will find as you continue to practice that your range will expand. You will notice the breath flowing evenly and the voice becoming smooth. You will also begin to hear the expression of emotions—anger, disappointment, joy—in your voice.

At times your chanting may be caressing, gentle, intense, full of longing or surrender. If you chant softly, you may observe that your emotions become more gentle. They will become refined through the chanting and change into true feelings which are expressed in the heart. At other times your voice may be strong and powerful as you put into it all your anger and disappointment, your requests and demands. Honestly express to God what you feel, even your anger and impatience toward the Divine for not bringing you sooner to the Light. But you must learn when to stop expressing emotions or your practice will become emotional self-indulgence.

When you find that your emotions are extremely difficult to control, you may give them back to the Divine. You may address the Divine at a very personal level, saying, "Why did You give me all these emotions? Why did You not give me the strength and insight to handle them? I want You to come here now and do something about it; open the door or pull the curtain back so that I can see why I feel this way." This may not seem like a form of prayer, but it is. It is the recognition of the need for help and the willingness to ask God for that help, and that is humility.

In chanting out the emotions, from the ugliest to the most exalted, and giving them back to the One who gave them to you in the first place, you learn to accept both parts of yourself, the good and the bad, and to transcend the pairs of opposites, from which we are trying to free ourselves. On the spiritual path, by channeling the emotions toward God, we find that the Divine accepts our struggle and aids and sustains us in our search for the Most High.

Emotions in themselves are not bad, but when running wild they can be extremely damaging. Even love, when not shared, not given freely and generously, becomes self-love which turns destructively back on the individual. When emotions are directed, they are a source of strength for great achievements. Through the power of emotions men and women have overcome their limitations and attained a higher purpose in life. Emotions channeled through a Mantra toward the Divine can take you close to God.

When chanting a Mantra the emotions express themselves in the breath and the voice. Every time the breath is uneven it means the emotions are involved and we are out of balance. As long as the emotions are running high, this imbalance exists, but gradually they subside and we begin to experience the equilibrium that is our goal. Then, as quietness descends, we can tune into the great rhythm of the Cosmos and become one with that rhythm. Chanting helps us to achieve this stillness by bringing the breath and the emotions under control. In these moments of complete stillness of the mind, indescribable bliss is experienced. By repeated practice it becomes possible to hold onto the contact made with our innermost being.

It is sad that most people can be single-pointed only when they are in distress. When they are joyful they are single-pointed for an instant, but then they begin to scheme to keep the joyful mood, and the scheming destroys it. But you can use the ability to be single-pointed in distress to let go and give back your emotions. You can say, "Well, I'm sorry, but I have to admit that I am like a baby that can't even walk. You must come and pick me up. You will have to wait until I can walk. And if You want me to walk, if You don't want me always to be a spiritual baby, then You must come now and help me." There comes a time when each seeker must take off the spiritual baby shoes, but for a while do not be too proud to be God's little child.

As the Mantra is chanted, moods will in time be brought under control and awareness in the here and now will grow. Attention, and therefore energy, will be withdrawn from the old thought patterns which, like tapes on a tape recorder, play over and over. These mental background noises keep us tied to the past and future, to fearful imaginings and senseless fantasies, which cause our self-created sufferings. The energy will now be channeled to the Most High, to a positive affirmation of one's inner-most Self.

The ability to concentrate, to achieve single-point-edness, and the overcoming of self-will go hand-in-hand. In the beginning, you may wonder, as I did, why you are sitting there chanting when you could be doing so many other things and helping so many people. These are typi-cal thoughts, typical complaints, as you go through a tug-of-war with your mind which wants to prevent your Higher Self from gaining control. Here "mind" and "ego" do not mean "pride" and "vanity." They refer rather to a body-mind which is the ruler in most people's lives. When the Higher Self is encouraged to exert mastery through the practice of Mantra Yoga, the many personality aspects which have ruled your life suddenly become apparent. These personality aspects, when threatened, put up a fight; they do not want to lose their hold.

Through the practice of Mantra and Japa Yoga you will find yourself in direct confrontation with the lower self, the ego or body-mind. You will become aware of those personality aspects that have been in control and have ruled your life. Now the Higher Self begins to take possession.

The ego or personality aspects of the intellectual will put up a greater fight than those of the rather naive per-son. The latter is more able to say, "Yes, I see where I was wrong; I won't do that again," while the intellectual is busy thinking up rational explanations to justify mistakes. There is often little humility in the intellectual. One of the dan-gers facing the follower of Jnana Yoga, the yoga of the mind, is that the practitioner may look down on practitioners of Bhakti Yoga, the yoga of love and devotion. This only in-dicates that the mind has not been used to develop true discrimination. Many swamis and yogis in India told me they hoped to be reincarnated as women in their next lives because women have true devotion, true humility, and this is the path to liberation.

To overcome the ego one must practice surrender. One must be able to surrender to the Mantra itself and to the energy of the Mantra. This requires purification. If you cannot surrender, that energy will feed the ego. Many disciples prostrate themselves at the feet of their Guru as an aid in developing humility. The disciple is, in fact, prostrating himself to the Divine Spirit that is in the Guru, and in all of us.

Learning to surrender to the Mantra and to the energy of the Mantra puts in motion the process of purification of the self, facing up to and eliminating selfishness, self-glorification, self-justification, and self-gratification. Do not let the intellectual mind distract you from attempting the practice of Mantra and Japa. No amount of words or book knowledge can give you the experience. You have to practice yourself for the effect to be understood.

If you go to bed at night and fall asleep with the Mantra, it will probably stay with you and you will wake up with it. You will not have dreams, because the generative power of the Mantra dissolves problems and removes the pressures that come from self-importance and self-will. If you fall asleep with the Mantra, you may make contacts that will eliminate your mental and verbal acrobatics about concepts of mind, self, and Cosmic Intelligence.

Because of its effect on the subconscious, people sometimes think that Mantra is a form of hypnotism. It is not possible to hypnotize yourself into becoming holy. There would be a deep conflict and either the mind would one day become deranged or you would go back to your old way of living.

It is important to reflect on hypnotism, however, because for many years we have been hypnotizing ourselves and have thereby set up limitations which prevent us from seeing and making use of our full potential. We are constantly bombarded through television with the idea that we must have a new car or that our bodies have odors which must be concealed. Researchers tell us that simply watching the television screen puts our brainwaves into those of a hypnotic trance pattern. Television, however, is only one of the most obvious means of hypnotism. In more subtle ways we are told throughout our lives that we must have a good job, make money, and be married. All this is hypnotism.

If we think, too, of reincarnation, we have to consider that for many lifetimes we have hypnotized ourselves into becoming what we are today, into the strong beliefs that have become prejudices. These prevent us from seeing the beauty and the truth of the Divine, not only in others, but in ourselves. The chanting of a Mantra, by focusing the mind on the name of God and the power of the Divine within our being, works to counteract these preconceptions. Mantra practice is actually a process of dehypnotizing because greater awareness and understanding are achieved, however slow the process may be.

We can become what we put into our minds, and therefore if we put the intense effort, the drive, and the power of the emotions into becoming a millionaire, we can probably achieve that. However, the same amount of energy can be put into becoming Self-Realized, and that is a goal truly worth the effort. After Realization there is very little left to wish for, but after one has become a millionaire there is a whole new set of problems and desires: how do I keep the money? how can I make more money? how will I find friends who love me for what I am and not for my money? But if one becomes Self-Realized then all are friends, because one can see the Divine in everyone.

Through the use of Mantra a greater sensitivity, a refinement of the senses, comes about which may eventually bring you to the point where you can see with the inner eye and hear with the inner ear. When the inner ear is developed, the music of the spheres may be heard, music of such exquisite beauty as no instrument, no human voice, is able to produce. The Cosmic AUM might be heard. The impact and effects of such experiences will bring an intense desire to change for the better.

Mantra is not a magic pill; rather it is like a steady stream of water which gradually wears down the hardest stone. The immediate results of chanting are an increase in the ability to concentrate, followed gradually by control of the breath and the emotions. Later the emotions will become refined into true feelings. The most important goal in chanting, however, is the Realization of the Self.

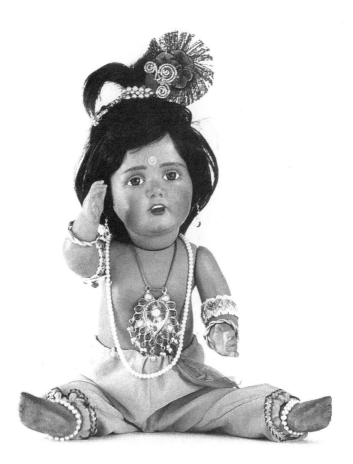

Baby Krishna

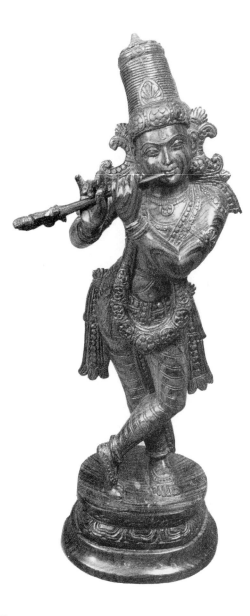

Krishna, the flute player

CHAPTER SIX

How to Use the Mantra

 Chanting is an individual matter and each person has a right to his or her own understanding. There can be no hard and fast rules. If you seek God, it is like a love affair between you and God. As you approach the Most High you grow and your understanding grows. You approach truth differently, gaining new perspective and insights.

The power of the Mantra becomes most effective when practiced regularly and for a sufficient period of time—that is, until you get results. How long you chant at one time or how frequently is your decision. You are working with the laboratory of your mind so you must allow a reasonable period of effort to give it a fair trial. You cannot become a saint in a weekend. It takes nine months for a baby to be born and many more years to grow into an adult; the beginner on the spiritual path is like a spiritual baby.

When you begin chanting you will find that a wave of enthusiasm carries you through the first period. Unfortunately, this soon passes as the mind wants a change, something new. Mantra practice is upsetting to the mind, forcing it out of its normal habits into a narrow path, making it single-pointed through discipline, and cutting the attachments to which it has clung. Like a child with new toys, the mind has a tendency to flit from one thing to another without discrimination. But the true reward will come only by perseverance and practice; only then will the secret of Mantra be discovered, its mystery and power revealed.

Awareness is essential; mere dreaming during the chanting will not "light the fire that consumes." Nor is it merely many hours of chanting or many thousands of repetitions or sheer will-power that lights this fire. The practice must be carried out with intensity. With application, with the purifying of the emotions, and with the mind more single-pointed, stillness will ensue and a sense of the ever-present Presence may be felt.

Combine formal Mantra practice with daily reflection and the keeping of a spiritual diary. This will help you to cultivate awareness and make the necessary changes in daily life to remove all aspects of egoism. Record the reactions of your mind to the practice and the obstacles encountered, as well as the changes you observe within yourself and any experiences you may have. It is by keeping a close watch throughout your practice that you will achieve a full understanding, not only of the Mantra, but also of the functioning of the mind. Knowing the impasses the mind encounters and also how it can overcome them can be very helpful in any situation in life.

After the first wave of enthusiasm for the practice of Mantra, there comes rebellion and opposition. The first critical point occurs at the end of two weeks, then three months, then two years. If you know the pattern ahead of time, you can take precautions. The mind is like an elephant. You cannot force an elephant to move rigidly along a fixed line. Rather you allow it to sway a little from side to side. You don't let it go sightseeing and forget its destination. Similarly, you can give the mind a little leeway but do not let it go entirely its own way.

One of the greatest problems in concentrating the human mind stems from the mental background noises. These are an accumulation of influences from the world around us, memories, and impressions which are triggered by the law of thought association. It is difficult to be completely quiet because we seem to be forever in the company of all these imprints which the mind has stored and turns out at random. When you first attempt to develop single-pointedness, you will become aware of this inability to keep the mind still. To deal with this, you can trick the mind into concentrating by the use of techniques which vary the practice without essentially changing the focus, techniques which allow the mind to be active within the framework of the Mantra.

You may, for example, think of all the details of chanting, how the sound is produced, the breathing, the effect of the sound on the body. An exercise such as this, although undertaken to maintain single-pointedness, can lead to many insights. You may also speed up the tempo of your chanting, including a greater number of repetitions within the span of one breath. Then slow it down, extending a name or syllable, stressing the first syllable, or the last. (This is dealt with more specifically in the section on *Hari Om* in Chapter Seven.) Vary the volume of the voice, first swelling the sound, then softening it. This kind of variety keeps the mind interested while still involving it fully and so helps to keep the repetitions from becoming mechanical.

You may notice that your voice becomes smoother as you chant, that you can sing as you never could before. Delight in these improvements and put into your mind positive thoughts that you want to reach God by means of your voice, that you wish to be an instrument of God's love, and that the Mantra you chant will be of help to those in need. In this way you are master of the situation rather than becoming the slave of intellectual doubts and false pride.

During chanting, emotions may arise that you are unaware of having. Tears may come which you have been holding back for many years. You must use discrimination to recognize tears of self-pity and deny yourself that indulgence. Sometimes the tears will be part regret and part joy—joy that the soul is at last on its way back home, regret that so many lifetimes have been wasted. Symbolically collect your tears, whatever their origin, and offer them to the Divine.

Watch the flow of your breath and its relation to emotions to understand the difference between expressing emotions and indulging in them. Indulgence indicates that you have become the victim of undisciplined emotions.

Realize also that we cannot control the emotions through sheer will-power, so when they are too strong, give them back to God, ask for help as a child asks its mother. At that moment, when you cry out from the depths of your being, you are most sincere and you are single-pointed in your anger, disappointment, or anguish. In doing this, you will experience true humility, perhaps for the first time. To express humility, you can see yourself as either God's child or God's servant. If you are the kind of person to whom pleasing others is important, be God's servant. Then the Divine is your master; please the Divine. Offer yourself as an instrument through which divine love can be expressed to others. As you try to become more pleasing to God, you will find that divine love comes to you through people, who are God's creation. If God can love you, everybody can love you.

The Mantra should be chanted or recited in some quiet place at a regular time each day, but it can also be chanted while you are doing other things, such as washing dishes, shovelling snow, or any other household task. These tasks are also good for self-purification. While you are doing these tasks, your concentration need not be on the space between the eyebrows. If you are washing dishes you cannot keep your concentration there, but you can hold the mental image of the power of the Mantra personified in a deity, and so spiritualize your tasks. You can listen to the sound of your voice and watch your breath. You can create a desire and a liking for the Mantra by thinking of what a Mantra is, what the mystery and power of a Mantra are, how you create sounds, what happens to them, and whether the energy of the sound you produce disappears when it can no longer be heard.

At some point you may wish to experiment by chanting your Mantra and watching your dreams. Do this for a definite length of time and allow a reasonable period for results to emerge.

If you repeat the Mantra while doing Hatha Yoga, you will be able to penetrate the deeper levels of the asanas. Try holding an asana while you chant mentally, becoming absorbed in what you are doing. Gradually you will become aware of the pranic flow in the body, the deeper aspects of the asana, and finally you will experience its mystical meaning.

Start with an asana that you are fairly comfortable in. Sit in the spinal twist, for example, and repeat *Om Namah Sivaya* ten times, first on one side and then on the other. Then you can go through your body and think, "How many bends are there in my body? What else is my body doing at this time besides bending?" From there you can make a thorough investigation, trying to understand the psychological and symbolic or spiritual meaning of each asana.

Try the peacock pose *(mayurasana)* as another example. The peacock is associated with vanity and showing off. The asana itself is said to be beneficial for removing toxins from the body. Just as the peacock kills snakes, this asana "kills" toxins.[1] Then there is also the peacock that is the vehicle for Lord Subramanya, and the peacock used in Christian iconography to represent the glory of heaven. Think also of the position of the asana, how you are balanced with the elbows pressed against the abdomen in the region of the navel. Then reflect on all the meanings of these suggestions.[2]

Chanting Mantra in a Hatha pose, however, is a separate practice from your Mantra practice which you do daily in a place especially set aside for that purpose.

If you have found your spiritual teacher or Guru, chant his or her name as an offering, an act of love. Channel the emotions by giving admiration and gratitude for the inspiration you have received. This offering and the recognition of the divine spirit within the Guru will aid in

---

1   B.K.S. Iyengar, *Light on Yoga*, rev. ed. (New York: Schocken Books, 1976), 284.

2   For full instruction on reflection in Hatha Yoga, see Swami Sivananda Radha, *Hatha Yoga:the Hidden Language*, (Spokane, WA, USA: Timeless Books, 1987).

developing humility and overcoming the ego. You may use the raga of a Mantra to do this.[3]

It will always help to listen to the Mantra. If you are working at something and cannot say the Mantra silently, or if you are very tired and do not feel that you have the will-power to sit and chant yourself, have the Mantra tape playing in the background. When you play a tape, always use the same Mantra; do not play a variety of tapes.[4]

Listening to a Mantra tape can also be a great help when you are going to sleep. If you watch the late news on television, everything you see or hear will be taken into your sleep and you may have nightmares. If there is negativity in what you read, this too may manifest in your sleep. Television watching and reading are done to satisfy the carnal mind and they need to be counteracted. If you have an argument before you go to bed, you will take the anger to bed with you and it, too, will manifest in your sleep. The unconscious will try to free itself of the emotion by working it out in a dream. Playing the Mantra tape as you are going to sleep will help to counteract all this. By continually playing the tape and chanting whenever you have a few moments to yourself, the habit of keeping the Mantra close to the surface in the day-to-day events of your life will gradually become stronger and will help to overcome the negativity of daily experience.

The length of your practice is an individual matter and will change from time to time. There really is no limit to either the length of time or the number of repetitions

---

3   Using a Mantra *raga* in this way can invoke the Guru's presence in the mind and heart, and does not have any adverse or negative effects, although it is not usually considered a traditional use of Mantra. Also, see the section on *Hari Om* in Chapter Seven.

4   A list of suitable tapes appears in the Bibliography.

you may chant. I once chanted five hours a day for two years. Later I continued to chant for only two hours, because by then I had built up what is called "mantric power," which is necessary before one can give another person a Mantra initiation. I chanted five hours because it took that long for my mind to become single-pointed. There have been spiritual giants in India who have chanted ten hours a day for many years. Obviously, the more you put into it, the more you will achieve. However, a few minutes of being absolutely with the Mantra is better than many hours of chanting if your mind is not focused. It is better, for example, to chant for ten minutes with concentration than for five hours with the mind wandering.

If you wish to chant Mantra do not worry if you do not know exactly how Sanskrit words are pronounced. When I asked Swami Sivananda how important the correct pronunciation was, he said, "Your sincerity and what is in your heart and mind are more important than your pronunciation. There are thousands of people who pronounce words correctly, but they have not yet become saints." It is your love of God, your persistence and devotion, and your intentions that will bring results, not correct pronunciation.

It is very important, however, to use the correct melody. Even if you find the higher notes difficult, you must not sing them an octave lower or change the key. Over time, the singing voice can be changed. Because it is important to sing the correct note at the correct pitch, my own music Guru at the Ashram in Rishikesh, Swami Nada Brahmananda, went to great trouble to help me increase the range of my voice.

If you wish to request blessings for friends and relatives, you may say their names aloud between repetitions of the Mantra, but you should not keep your mind on the individuals. Your concentration should remain on the Mantra itself, the different tones, or the image of the deity connected with it. Do not think of the image of the person for whom you are chanting, because by doing that you may interfere with that person and this you must not do.

If you realize after your practice that your mind and heart were not really in it, offer it to the Divine, saying, "You are the loving God of which I am created. This is all I could do today." You cannot always be one hundred percent in your practice, but you must try, and you must have the honesty and humility to admit it to yourself and to the Most High whenever you fall short.

Tape your voice occasionally when you chant, and date the tape. You can follow your own development by listening to the sound of your voice three months later, or a year or ten years later. Make a note of the emotions you experienced and listen for them in your voice on the tape.

When the practice of Mantra goes on for several hours at a stretch, mental chanting (Manasika) and the various other forms of Japa can be alternated in order to maintain concentration. Mental repetition is considered by some yogis the most powerful form, but for many people the audible chanting is more successful while the mind is still very active because it helps to express emotions. At a much later stage the mental repetition will be found more potent. Sometimes it is a good idea to recite the Mantra mentally when you are in the presence of others. This will restrain the urge to show off. When the awareness of this desire arises, say "Thank you," because such awareness will increase when gratitude is felt.

Another variation you may use is Likhita Japa, in which the Mantra is written down in lines like sentences, or in shapes and forms, as in the diagram of a lotus, or a cross, or in any design that will help to reinforce your devotions. One uniform system of writing will help concentration. If you work in an office, it is an excellent way of using any free time for your spiritual development, rather than wasting it in socializing. Writing the Mantra may also be alternated with other forms of Japa to maintain the focus on the Mantra, while providing variation to keep the mind interested. Keep all sheets of paper or notebooks in which you have written the Mantra near your bed or on your altar, because they have a very subtle effect on the subconscious.

The Mantra may be recited rather than sung, but the voice must be clear and intense enough that the ears may pick up what is being said. Bring the mind to the questions: What does this Mantra mean to me today? Does this ancient practice have any validity in today's world? This will help you remain fully engaged and focused on the Mantra.

You may find that different forms of Japa are effective at different times. Whatever form you are using, take the first few minutes of your practice to get the mind in order, to focus the feelings and emotions on what you are doing. Then direct all your efforts to the glorification of God, expressing your feelings of gratitude for having received knowledge of this practice and being able to help yourself. This attitude may not always be possible for you. If it is not, acknowledge your negativity and offer it to the Divine. Remember that being involved with God, even in anger, is better than being lukewarm or indifferent.

Later, when the practice is established, you will find that inspiration, the answers to your prayers, will come when you have finally surrendered, when you have chanted or repeated the Mantra to the point that the mind is exhausted. It is like being a scientist in the laboratory, who tries and tries, only to find that inspiration comes when at last the reasoning mind is exhausted.

If, after a year or two of practice, there emerges by itself a different way of practicing Mantra Yoga, it should not be suppressed. This may be guidance from a higher level. But make sure it is not the ego wanting to have its own way. First do your practice the way you have been taught and see what the results are. Then allow yourself to try the new way and see if the same results can be reached. If changes are made too soon, based on assumption rather than experience, the results cannot be obtained. Dig one deep well rather than many shallow ones. Only when, through expanding awareness, you realize that one lesson is completed, are you ready to move on to another.

If you are completely serious in your efforts, you may reach a time when you want to do an extended Mantra practice. This will bring steadily deepening God-communion and release from emotional imbalance, bringing the self into harmony with the Self.

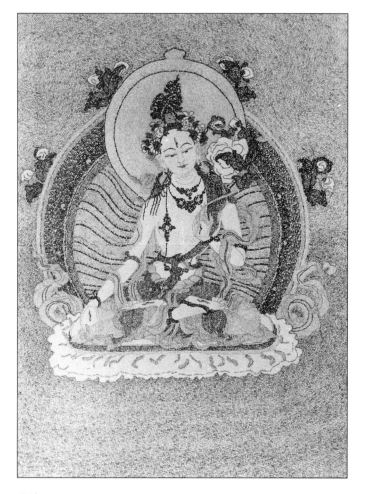

White Tara (Likhita Japa)

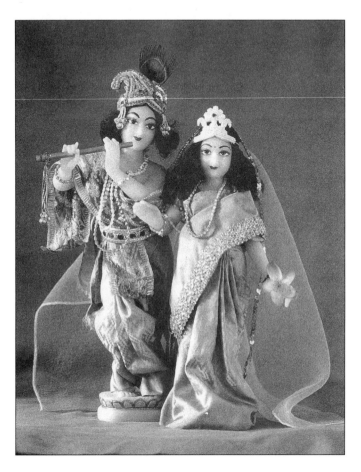

*R*adha and Krishna

CHAPTER SEVEN

Individual Mantras

 The Mantras presented in the first section of this chapter are Mantras of the heart, used as short formulas to bring about single-pointedness of mind for the purpose of achieving Self-Realization. Toward the end of the chapter, there are other examples of Mantras you may wish to chant for other purposes, as well as suggestions on chanting other texts.

Most Mantras are associated with an aspect of the Divine. This gives the mind something to work with. The mind is creative; as soon as you give it some material it weaves a pattern all its own. When you begin to chant, it immediately creates an image or symbol of the Divine, usually as a super-human being, because this is the only way the mind can understand Cosmic Energy as a power that will take a personal interest in human beings. It is important that the image created have meaning for you as an individual, that it sum up what is to you the best, most beautiful, most perfect divine love. This image is your mind in its most creative aspect.

However, this creation can be easily mistaken during chanting as coming from some higher divine source. You may fall in love with your creation and forget that it is only your creation. Then this image becomes the rival of God in your mind.

The advantage of not knowing what the Mantra means is that the mind has nothing to work on. Then, when the Mantra does reveal itself to you, there is no doubt of its meaning. However, although an intellectual explanation encompasses only a small part of the Mantra's significance, knowing the meaning, while understanding the creativity of the mind, may hasten the revelation.

There are many Mantras because there are many different kinds of people. There is a particular sound or vibration to which your spiritual body will best respond, and so there is a Mantra especially suited to you, but this does not mean that no one else will have the same Mantra. However, the Mantras are not so different as they may appear. *Hari Om,* a Mantra to invoke Lord Krishna, is not so different from *Om Namah Sivaya* as it may appear to the beginner. Both lead to an understanding of the greater Oneness but by different approaches. Krishna is like a lover luring the devotee into a personal relationship with the Divine by the haunting sound of his flute. Here the devotee is led by an inclination to romance into a partnership with Krishna, thereby easing feelings of loneliness. Siva may appeal to a devotee who ardently wishes to overcome some obstacles on the spiritual path. Here the devotee may appeal for help and protection.

Each Mantra will lead to God-Realization, to the top of the spiritual mountain, but each one will take a slightly different path. In each situation the natural inclinations and temperament of the devotee are met. Is that not what we see everywhere in life? Each person is drawn to that which he or she finds most attractive, desirable, and satisfying. The division between the power and the meaning of Mantras will disappear as the spiritual aspirant matures. The understanding of Eastern psychology takes on greater and greater subtlety until the aspirant is finally no longer dependent on the personal aspect of that awesome power called by these various names.

To choose your own Mantra, you can listen to tapes giving samples of several Mantras.[1] One way to make a choice is to stretch out in a comfortable position with closed eyes, listen to the tape, and see if there is any intuitive response to a particular Mantra. If there is, then that is the Mantra to choose.

In the course of time another Mantra may come to the surface quite naturally. The melody may just come up by itself. You should make detailed inquiries into this, to ascertain that the appearance of this new Mantra is not just due to the restlessness of the mind. You should not change to another Mantra until you have some experience of the power of the first one. It is not until a later stage of development, when several Mantras have become active within you, that you can use several simultaneously. You must start with one Mantra and lay a good foundation. Then, when your comprehension has grown and you understand that all power is indeed one, there is no confusion. You can take another Mantra and chant it to know the difference in experience. Then when you want to help others, you will be able to help them from many angles.

---

1   See list of tapes in Bibliography.

AUM

The Cosmic sound *AUM,* or its condensed form *OM,* is the origin of all other sounds and is itself a Mantra. It is called the *Pranava,* or sacred syllable, and symbolizes Brahman or the essential spiritual reality. The Mantra *AUM* gives birth to rays of Light, bringing illumination to the mind.

All sounds are blended into the beautiful Cosmic *AUM,* which can reverberate in the hearts of men and women. Mantra is speech most profound, sound at its purest, and when that supreme sound of *OM* becomes sovereign, it takes you past the little selfish ego, so that you are clothed in new cloth of thought and sound. You will be lifted beyond all other existence and when you speak, you will hear the sound of the Self, your innermost Being.

The flute of Lord Krishna is also symbolic for the Pranava. By the sound of his flute, Krishna created the world, and with its sound, he calls his devotees back to their heavenly home. Like the flute, the devotee must be empty, with egoism and self-importance removed. In that perfect and complete surrender, the mortal aspect, the self-will, becomes merged with the Divine and blends in joy and harmony, producing a sound of great inspiration, the cosmic sound of *AUM.* Swami Sivananda has said that in this kind of self-surrender, which comes from the very core of one's heart, spiritual practice or *sadhana* is not necessary, because one has truly become the Lord's property, the flute of Lord Krishna.

AUM must be chanted in three parts, with equal time given to each part; *Ah* is chanted in the region of the navel, *00* in the sternum, and *MM* in the throat.

Here is an example of a meditation you can use,

which can help you to gain understanding and insights into this Mantra, and which can help you develop your own meditation. When you chant *Ah,* place the sound at the navel or solar plexus. Visualize a lotus representing life itself. See a fluctuation of Light energy on its petals. Imagine a change in color from bright red to that of rain clouds. Allow these fluctuations to move, almost as if they have a life of their own. Think of them as symbolic for changing moods. Now see the tips of the lotus petals become faint pink, then let the lotus gradually become a shimmering white. Think of this as the Divine Light of insights, understanding, and love dispersing the rain clouds of ignorance.

As the Light expands, let the next lotus, the heart center, come into focus. Chant *OO* and place the sound at the area of the sternum. See the petals of this lotus as red at the center and pink in the middle, with the tips becoming clear white. As you chant, think of how refined the emotions can become when cultivated by such practices as this.

When the last sound, *MM,* is chanted with closed lips, you will become aware of your physical response and the vibration of the many, many cells of your body. When you chant, listen with great attention and contemplate the innate power of sound and its ability to manifest. This will lead to hearing the Cosmic *AUM* which is not a physical experience, but one that is heard by the inner ear, always the right. *M* becomes symbolic for surrender and for the response of the body as it reverberates to Pranavanada, the sound of the Most High.

The chanting of *AUM* will purify the mind, destroy all evil, all egoism. *AUM* represents the trinity of the physical, mental, and spiritual bodies; waking consciousness, dream consciousness, and dreamless sleep; and also individual, universal, and transcendental consciousness.

Listening to the sound of Lord Krishna's flute, all consciousness is submerged in the Divine. Listening to the reverberations of the *AUM* within, the devotee becomes divine. In the chanting of *AUM* one empties oneself and is filled with an essence that is beyond description.

KRISHNA INVOCATION

The name of Krishna may be invoked and used as a Mantra. The *Krishna Invocation* contains an allegorical story with the sequence of notes resembling the crying of a child for its father or mother. The devotee is a child of the Divine, and just as the child calls out for its parent, the devotee cries for God in the manifestation of Lord Krishna. Krishna may also be seen as the Cosmic Lover, or as the Oversoul, with the singer as the soul in search of the Lord.

This Mantra begins at a low tone and works up gradually, like the child who does not get an immediate response, until there is the realization that attention cannot be commanded of either the parent or of God. Then there is resignation as the voice drops. But soon the demands start again with strength and energy, feelings and emotions. Just as the human mother or father knows and responds only to the real cry for help, so God pays little attention to us as long as we are caught up with our worldly toys and games—cars, houses, position, achievements.

The devotee must learn that Lord Krishna cannot be commanded, and will not produce a vision or spiritual experience at the individual's convenience. When there is surrender to the fact that the Divine comes in its own time, and when the flood of uncontrolled emotions is cleared away, only then in that silence there may come a response.

This Mantra is a devotional fire that consumes the emotional dross, brings the heart to pure longing, the mind to stillness, and the soul to peace.

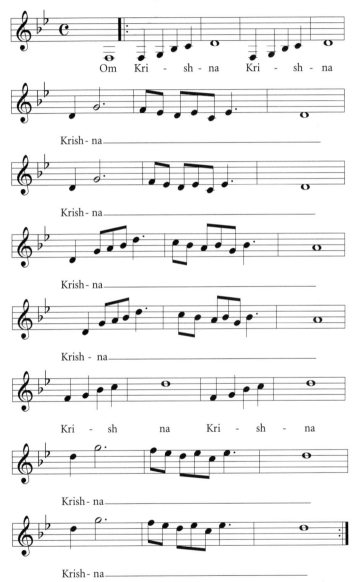

OM KRISHNA GURU

Om Krishna Guru is especially helpful if you are seeking a teacher. Its practice can bring you to your Guru.

The Mantra begins with *Om*, the Supreme Energy, beyond all names and forms, the essence of all energy. *Krishna* is this energy manifest which is shaped and formed by the human mind for its own convenience. We all create God in our own image. For example, Jesus, the man, the Middle Easterner, was probably swarthy-skinned and dark-haired, yet he is often portrayed as blond and blue-eyed. This image is a creation of the mind. It is thus that we personalize the impersonal power, and so such images as Siva, Krishna, Tara, and Jesus are all creations of the human mind, manifestations of the Supreme Energy. If you want to love God, you can only love that power when it manifests as creation. Loving God means loving people, loving plants, loving animals, loving all that you think of as God's creation. This may be difficult, but we can begin by having reverence for life in all its forms.

Lord Krishna is always shown standing when he plays the flute, his body making a cross. This means that he is lenient with human frailties, but it also symbolizes the control of the three gunas of this world. Very often he is shown standing on a lotus or with one flowering near him. The lotus is untainted by the muddy water in which it grows; the inner Light of every human being is untainted; the universe is untainted. The dark blue color of Krishna signifies the unknown; although Krishna is in human form, the Divine can never be known in its entirety.

Guru is the spiritual teacher, the one who dispels our ignorance and brings us to the Light.

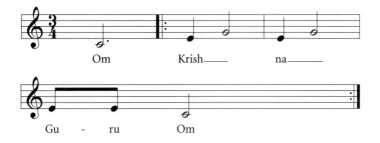

Om   Krish——   na——

Gu - ru   Om

RADHE GOVINDA

Radhe Govinda is a charming representation of emotions and the spiritual search, and of the relationship between Divine Energy as personified by Krishna and its manifestation as personified by Radha. *Govinda* means "the one who tends the cows" and is another name for Lord Krishna. *Radha*, through her unceasing love for God, is the symbol of humanity eternally seeking the Divine.

When love has become Cosmic, it no longer has a "because" attached to it. The human relationship can have these divine qualities when the love for God obliterates self-centeredness. The story of this Mantra, like the Krishna Invocation, displays an understanding of human nature and an acceptance of it as the vehicle through which we reach the Divine.

Radha calls for Krishna and they play a game of hide-and-seek. Krishna withdraws, Radha searches. He returns, but keeps disappearing and reappearing. Radha becomes bored and drops the search; she is distracted and petulant. Now it is Krishna's turn to take the initiative and win

Radha over. This is to reveal and to illustrate the sublime truth that God loves the devotee at least as much as the devotee loves God.

The chanting of the *Radhe Govinda* Mantra should be infused with the most intense feelings of love. It should be sung with the God-centered aspiration to find the Divine within, which deepens that love, and to find God in all humankind, which broadens that love.

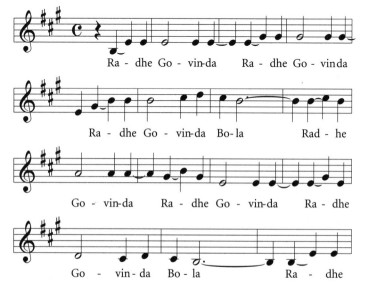

Ra - dhe Go - vin-da Ra - dhe Go - vin-da

Ra - dhe Go - vin-da Bo- la Rad - he

Go - vin-da Ra - dhe Go - vin-da Ra - dhe

Go - vin - da Bo - la Ra - dhe

OM TARA

In the Tibetan Buddhist tradition, Divine Mother is known as *Tara*. As the White Tara, she represents the highest intelligence of the Buddha, the All-Knowing One. The Buddha is often shown in her crown. The White Tara has seven eyes: one in each of her hands and feet, the third eye in the

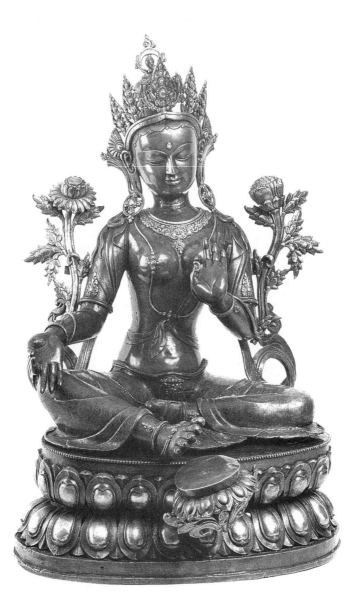

Tara, granter of boons

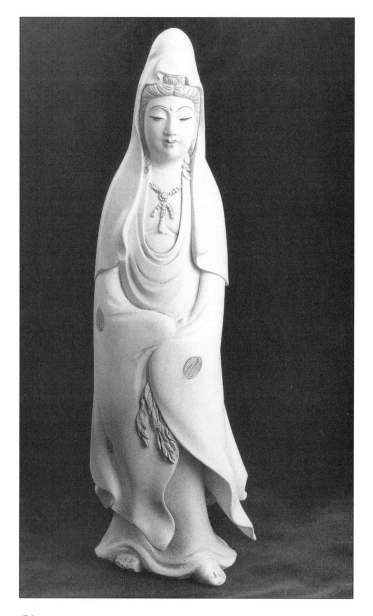

Kuan Yin, goddess of compassion

center of her forehead, and the two that all human beings have. These symbolize clearly her All-Seeing Eye, or a power of clairvoyance that is beyond our imagination.

As the Green Tara, she is the Mother of Compassion. She may be called upon as a child calls to its mother for she is ever ready to come to the rescue of her devotees.

Tara means "star." For thousands of years, ships have been navigated at night by using the stars. Tara is the guiding star showing the way to the other shore. In the interplay of the gaseous forces in a star, however, there is a great devouring power, and Tara has also the aspect of Kali who devours her creation. In our personal life as we seek the Most High, time devours us. So Tara is also a symbol of time, which must not be wasted.

This Mantra helps us to develop an understanding that our lives, the world and all it contains are nothing other than the manifestation of divine power. Chanting *Om Tara* puts us in touch with the ever-present reality of divine manifestation and can lead us beyond it.

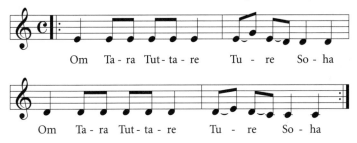

AVE MARIA

Ave Maria, although not a Mantra in the Indian tradition, has gained enormous power through the countless repetitions of the Christians who have chanted it. *Ave Maria* is part of the much longer Hail Mary prayer of which these two words are the essence. I have presented it here as part of a short prayer with a melody to which it may be sung. When used in the way that a Mantra is used, *Ave Maria* will produce results similar to those achieved through the chanting of traditional Indian Mantras. In Hindu mythology and religious thought the female principle is seen as the creative power through which the universe is manifested. In Christian terms, *Ave Maria,* the Hail Mary, is the worship of the mother, the love aspect of the Divine. This brings out the noblest feelings in the human being. In Hindu teachings, the seeker can approach the ultimate spirit of God, which is beyond all manifestation, only through the mother principle of the manifested universe. The devotee who wants to enter the house of the Lord has first to go to Divine Mother for the keys—love and devotion—before entry can be attained.

Ave Maria creates a deep feeling of love for the Divine. It will bring you in contact with Divine Mother herself. Dedicate the chanting to those whom you wish to bless.

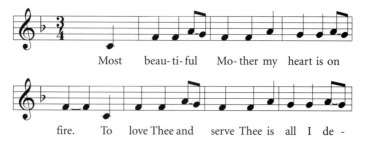

Most beau-ti-ful Mo-ther my heart is on fire. To love Thee and serve Thee is all I de -

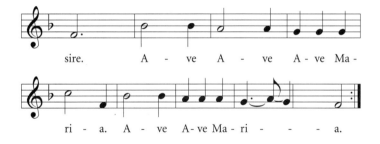

sire. A - ve A - ve A - ve Ma -

ri - a. A - ve A- ve Ma - ri - - - a.

HARI OM

Hari Om is the healing Mantra. *Hari* is a name for Vishnu, the preserving aspect of the Divine. Krishna is also an aspect of the preserving or sustaining force, and so Hari may be thought of as the healing aspect of Lord Krishna. God assumes many aspects in order to provide us with a variety of ways to tackle our difficulties, according to individual characteristics and temperament.

In Sanskrit, *Hari* means "to take away." Vishnu takes away the consequences of offences, errors, and follies, when there is repentance. These are the impurities that bring about grief and sickness. If they are removed, health and strength are conserved for spiritual endeavors.

Om or AUM is the Hindu trinity, which here means creation, preservation, and destruction: the generation within us of that which is pure, sacred, and noble; the sustaining and strengthening of these qualities; and the dissolving of all that is impure and negative.

This Mantra calls on Vishnu (or Lord Krishna) to preserve the human body and the mind in the best state of health for the purpose of finding Self-Realization, attaining to the Om, the Cosmic concept that absorbs all aspects in One, finally becoming formless.

The *Hari Om* Mantra is most powerful between midnight and three o'clock in the morning. At this time worldly vibrations are calm and mental activity is less. This is the time at which you are most likely to have a spiritual experience.

Since the science of sound and breath control applies to any religion, Christians can chant *Jesus Christ* to the tune of *Hari Om*, while Jews can use *Adonai* or *Elohim*. A Buddhist might choose one of the names of Lord Buddha; or you can chant the words, *Divine Mother,* or use any one of her 108 names, such as Radha, Lakshmi, or Saraswati. When a spontaneous feeling of gratitude wells up toward your teacher or Guru, this may be expressed by using the teacher's name as a way of blessing and giving thanks for all that has been received. You can go from one to another of these names, in order to give greater variety to the chanting, without changing the notes and the key in which the Mantra is sung.

Through the various ways in which it can be chanted, *Hari Om* is effective in efforts to make the mind single-pointed. To control the restlessness of the mind and overcome feelings of doubt, changes may be made by stressing syllables or sounds differently, while keeping the melody the same. Here are some possibilities:

  * Sing in a soft voice, using normal breath to bring the mind slowly under control.

  * Sing a full sequence of Mantra in one breath, so the concentration is again gathered, like light through a magnifying glass, to become single-pointed and returned to the Mantra. Continue chanting for as long as you can keep the concentration single-pointed. If the mind begins

to behave like a monkey, jumping here and there, it is time to make another change.

    * Chant two sequences in one breath. This will again help to bring concentration back to the Mantra. When concentration begins to wane it is time to attempt three Mantras in one breath.

    * When thoughts crowd in and you cannot keep them out by any effort of will, try another change. Express your distress by emphasizing the *ee* sound in Hari.

    * Stress the *Ha*, with emphasis on the breath and tension of the muscles in the region of the solar plexus. Link this with the mind and throw out everything that is negative.

    * Another variation is to stress the *Om*, extending the sound as long as possible.

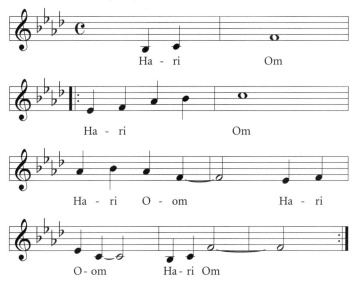

OM NAMAH SIVAYA

In *Om Namah Sivaya* the devotee appeals to God in the aspect of destroyer of all ignorance and illusion that stands in the way of the divine union. We need assistance in our efforts to overcome the ego. Self-centeredness cannot be mastered by sheer will-power; we must surrender and ask for divine help. *Om Namah Sivaya* is a call upon God to eliminate our negative qualities, to dissolve our difficulties, and to destroy the obstacles to higher spiritual life. Siva is called "The Compassionate One," removing such obstacles as selfishness and jealousy which impede our development. Lord Siva's destruction is really a blessing.

We must be prepared to have our concepts destroyed, as well as our preconceived ideas, and even our relationships. What we believe to be true and unshakeable today may be meaningless tomorrow. Some of our obstacles may be things to which we are very strongly attached. In seeking higher values, we have to ask, "Am I willing to pay the price?" The Most High is a pearl of great price. Attachment, whether to possessions, to fame, or to another individual, stands between the devotee and God.

Sometimes blessings come in disguise. An illness gives us time to be holy, time to think and to reflect on the purpose and direction of our life. Destruction on any level means turmoil and this is especially true on the spiritual level. But the old must be destroyed to make way for the new and in chanting this Mantra the devotee is asking Siva to perform this kind of destruction.

However, a mistake can be made in concentrating on the destructive aspect without invoking a feeling of gratitude that help is being given to overcome the obstacles. This involves two important human emotions: humility, to recognize that one needs help; and gratitude that, whenever it is sincerely asked for, this help is given. Imagine yourself driving along a road that has many potholes. Then someone appears ahead of you and begins filling in the holes. You would stop concentrating on the holes and instead feel grateful to the person who is filling them.

It is helpful to have a picture or image of Siva in your room and put fresh white flowers in front of it. The image of Lord Siva, sitting still and in silence on Mount Kailas in the snowy regions of the Himalayas, is a symbol for the state of complete silence and motionlessness which follows the destruction of emotional attachments and fears.

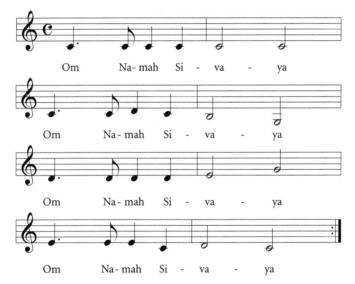

OM SRI RAMA JAYA RAMA

Om Sri Rama Jaya Rama Jaya Jaya Rama is a call to victory for the spiritual Self. *Rama* means one who delights in the consciousness of the spiritual Self. *Jaya* means "hail" or "victory." Rama represents the aspect of God as king and ruler of the universe. Chant this Mantra if you want to be God's servant, to carry out the divine will, and accept the Divine as king. It is used to evoke the power that leads to victory for the spiritual Self, that it may obtain realization of the Divine within.

Papa Ramdas, a saint of modern India, concentrated his search for God-Realization in the chanting of the *Ram* Mantra. He initiated all his devotees into the name of Ram, and had a deep relationship with God in the aspect of Ram. He talked to Ram and in moments of danger would ask, "Now, Ram, how are you going to save me? Or are you going to destroy me?"

Although not a literal translation, the words "I am Thine, all is Thine, Thy Will be done, O Lord" are in the spirit of the Mantra. While they are not true Mantra, they are an example of following inner inspiration and intuition to give the meaning in a different language and may be chanted as you would chant a phrase from the Bible.

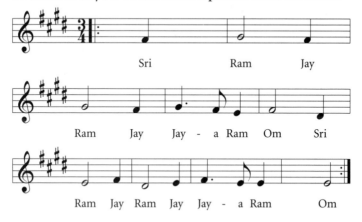

Sri Ram Jay
Ram Jay Jay - a Ram Om Sri
Ram Jay Ram Jay Jay - a Ram Om

* * *

Traditionally, the meaning of Mantras is not explained. It is by chanting the Mantra that the aspirant discovers the meaning. I am including here two Mantras without explanation so that anyone who wishes to do so may chant one of them until the meaning or power of the Mantra reveals itself.

NAMO AMITABHA

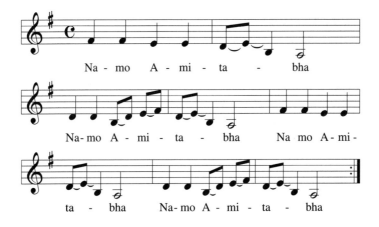

Na - mo A - mi - ta - bha

Na- mo A - mi - ta - bha Na mo A - mi -

ta - bha Na- mo A - mi - ta - bha

OM NAMO BAGHAVATE

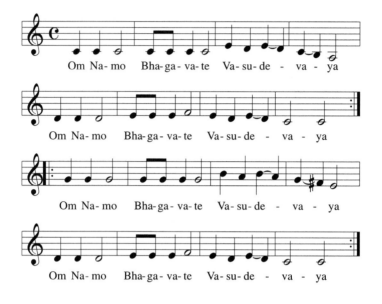

* * *

There are other types of Mantra which are not used directly to achieve Self-Realization. For example, the verses of the *Ananda Lahari* by Sankara of the first century C.E.[2] promise power or material benefits. They are mainly a description and glorification of the Hindu Divine Mother. The verses usually consist of four lines. The words are recited rather than chanted to a raga and they may be recited in a monotone to set them apart from daily chatter. Each verse has a specific yantra (abstract representation of the Divine).

---

2 *Ananda Lahari,* translation and commentary by Swami Sivananda, 4th ed. (Rishikesh: Divine Life Society, 1949).

In these Mantras, Divine Mother's power is invoked on many levels: one verse may be recited to gain the power to foresee the future through dreams; another may bring immunity from famine and pestilence; still others will remove sterility, cure consumption, or charm snakes.

Most have to be recited a thousand times a day for between thirty-five and forty-five days. This can take between eight and ten hours daily. The struggle to carry on after three or four days or a week is sometimes quite difficult. The mind may become as rebellious as a wild horse. Some people will go up and down several times, and then all of a sudden have a breakthrough so that they never again have any trouble with long periods of Mantra practice. The success of such practice lies in the process of purification.

Two Mantras of this kind are of particular help on the spiritual path. One is addressed to Divine Mother; the other is the ancient Mantra from the Divine Light Invocation.

THE DIVINE MOTHER MANTRA

O Divine Mother, may all my speech and
idle talk be Mantra,
All actions of my hands be mudra,
All eating and drinking be the offering of
oblations unto Thee,
All lying down prostrations before Thee.
May all pleasures be as dedicating my
entire self unto Thee.
May everything I do be taken as Thy worship.

This is a Mantra expressing the devotee's desire to be Divine Mother's handmaiden. It is said to bring knowledge of all the scriptures if repeated one thousand times a day for forty-five days, but if your mind is still full of psychological obstructions, or if your chanting has been mechanical, you will not achieve results.

You do not need to do such a lengthy practice, however, to have benefits from this Mantra. You may recite it five times a day for a week every three or four months. With the first line decide that you truly want your speech to be worthy of being considered as Mantra. Ask for help. At the end of the day, ask yourself, "What did I say today? Can I really offer what I have said to other people as Mantra?" Note your reflections in your spiritual diary. Next, think of how you use your hands each day and whether you are using them in Divine Mother's service. When you are eating, ask yourself for what purpose you are nourishing your body. What will you do with the energy from the food? Ask what other forms of nourishment there are. Reflect also that life is not only work; there are the pleasures of life as well. Offering all that you are, including the pleasures, will help free you from making mistakes. At the beginning of the day, ask that everything you do be worthy of offering as worship. At the end of the day, reflect to find out where you succeeded and where more effort is needed.

Sometime lie down on your back on the floor or outside and look at the ceiling or the sky. Imagine the most detailed image of Divine Mother; then project this image onto the ceiling or sky. Here is a lovely prayer I have often recited which may help you create an image.

Sakti, your body is the World.
The rivers are your veins,
And the forest, your hair.
The firmament is your dress.
The mind is your breath.
You are the pairs of opposites,
You are the past and the present,
The soft and the gentle,
The terrible and the fierce,
Your sounds are silence,
You are waves of sound,
And the power of silence,
You are the human and the Divine.
You are elevated places,
The labyrinth,
The one without a second.
O Mother of many aspects.

THE DIVINE LIGHT INVOCATION MANTRA

I am created by Divine Light.
I am sustained by Divine Light.
I am protected by Divine Light.
I am surrounded by Divine Light.
I am ever growing into Divine Light.

The words of the Divine Light Invocation may be used alone as a Mantra to help you identify with the Light and break negative attachments.[3] Reflect on each line. What does it mean to be created by Divine Light? What references to Light are there in other spiritual traditions? Visualize Light in a way that is meaningful to you—as a candle flame, a tiny spark, a roaring fire, the sun. Ask yourself how you use the cosmic energy that is within you. You may find when you do these reflections that they mean something different to you each day.

Light sustains. There is no life in a body without Light. Use your enthusiasm to fuel the Light. Let the Light protect you when you are frightened or worried; use it as protection against your own monkey-mind. You are surrounded by Divine Light. There is a divine being in everyone around you. Put everyone you talk to into the Light, even your pets.

The last line, "I am ever growing into Divine Light" is not part of the original Mantra. It came to me in a moment of inspiration and I added it because it expressed exactly what I wanted to do.

You may recite this Mantra taking one breath for the first two lines, another for the next two, and another for the final line. Take a breath between, and begin again.

* * *

---

3 For the full practice of the Divine Light Invocation, see Swami Sivananda Radha, *The Divine Light Invocation*, 3rd ed. (Spokane, WA, USA: Timeless Books, 1990).

BIBLICAL PHRASES

If you wish to repeat biblical phrases or affirmations, and if you are persistent in repeating them, you will achieve results because you will develop single-pointedness of mind, and the constant repetition of these phrases will fill your being with positive thoughts. These will help you to erase the negativity that you have allowed to accumulate over the years. You may not receive any outside help in the same way that you would if you were to chant a Mantra such as *Hari Om.* But that is not certain, because if your devotion is sincere and you continue your practice, God is sure to hear you.

THE LORD'S PRAYER

The Lord's Prayer is too long to be a Mantra, and there are too many different ideas within it, so you could not achieve single-pointedness. For example, first there is the statement, "Our Father, who art in heaven." Then there is a request, "Give us this day our daily bread." These induce a variety of thoughts, feelings, and emotions, leading us away from true single-pointedness. However, there are benefits to be obtained from reciting this prayer repeatedly and reflecting on the meaning of its parts. If the repetition is done with sincerity and meaning, it will bring your mind to a kind of concentration.

At one time, I did a practice of repeating the Lord's Prayer for many hours a day and reflecting on the meaning of its different parts. I gained many insights. I realized, for example, that "Give us this day our daily bread" does not refer just to the bread we eat or even to spiritual bread. "Bread" can refer to anything that may happen to you, both positive and negative. For example, if you were to have an overpowering experience of the Christ Consciousness, it could be terrifying if you did not know what it was. Unless you make a very special effort to extend the perception of your senses, you can absorb only so much. So when you ask that you may receive your daily bread, ask also that you not be given more than you can handle, or that you be given additional strength and perception to meet whatever comes your way. If reflected on this way, individually, each phrase of the Lord's Prayer can lead to single-pointedness.

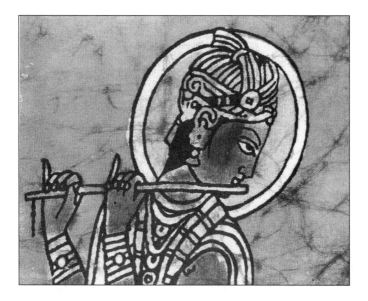

Krishna lures the devotee with his flute (batik)

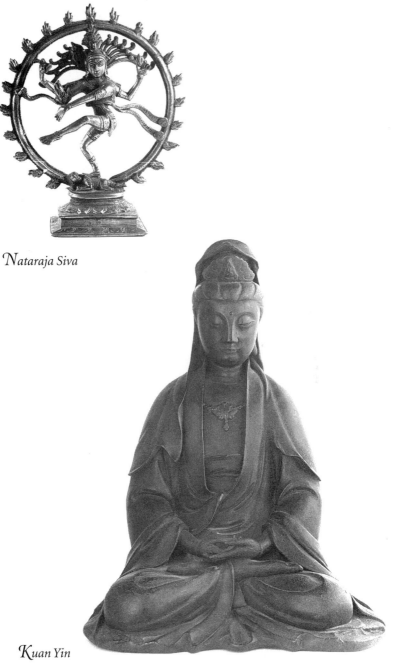

Nataraja Siva

Kuan Yin

CHAPTER EIGHT

Mantra & Healing

 There are many theories concerning healing, but your own observation and your own growing understanding will bring your own unique insights. With our limited minds, functioning only on the three-dimensional plane, we cannot really grasp all the law of the Divine, or the extended law of nature, nor understand the complicated causes of illness.

However, by chanting or praying with single-pointedness of mind, by reinforcing that concentration with action, by directing the will, healing will take place naturally within ourselves. Mantras can have a healing effect by releasing the emotions and bringing about a state of calmness and deep relaxation both in the chanter and in anyone listening. With the mind relaxed, the source of the disease and the hidden roots of conflict may come to the surface where they can be dealt with. But we must know why we want to be healthy, what we will do with the remainder of life if health is restored. We must be single-pointed in our desire. There may be advantages to being ill which, although we might not admit them consciously, our ego wants to hold onto. By enforcing our will and giving strength to that part which wants to be well, this polarity of the mind can be overcome, permitting healing to take place.

There is a Mantra, *Aham Brahmasmi*, which means "I am Brahman" or "I am God." This may seem a strange thought but a person becomes what she or he thinks. If you think you are a failure, you will become a failure. Conversely, if you continually chant *Aham Brahmasmi* you will eventually realize your divine nature and there will be little room for sickness at any level—physical, emotional, or mental. If you are to chant this Mantra, it is important that you clarify in your own mind what the meaning of God is to you. You must also do serious self-purification, and the other areas of your life must reflect this purification. You must develop the ability to surrender to the Mantra and to the energy that comes from it. You must have the humility to be able to ask for forgiveness and apologize to others if you are in the wrong.

Besides the ego's need for attention which perpetuates illness, and lack of humility which indicates a wrong attitude, there are many other factors which may interfere when you do spiritual practices for your own healing. You may have a lesson to learn, and so healing may not be what is best for you; you may be eating the wrong food, you may be exposed to a toxic environment, or you may be violating certain laws of nature to which your body is subject. You may hold an unhealthy belief that you are too great a sinner to deserve to be healed. You may also be hurting others without being aware of it and unconsciously punishing yourself for their pain. The complexity of the human mind and its capacity for pain is so tremendous that we must beware of over-simplification. Pain is a great teacher, but we must understand its message and deal with that before the way is clear for health to be restored.

All this must be remembered also in regard to the healing of others. It may be necessary for the person to experience pain or go through an illness in order to have the time to reflect, to develop humility and devotion, and to overcome selfishness. Perhaps a physical healing can take place only after the mind has been healed. You cannot know the purpose of an ailment, or its possible cause, nor can you know what is best for the person. But you may offer a prayer or chant Mantra, letting the power of the Mantra itself work. Chanting can be an expression of your sincere concern, although you must not decide how this help should be given.

When you chant or recite a Mantra for someone, visualize that person well and healthy. Do not picture the individual in a sick state, as such an image has remarkable power. Instead, invoke the image of Tara or Krishna or Siva or Jesus and, in full expectation, see the person standing in the radiance of Light. Let the healing force flow *through* you, never *from* you, and think of the energy of the Mantra as that healing Light. Wrap the individual in a spiral of this Light so that he or she becomes barely visible and let the image of this spiral move to the source of all Light.[1] Now focus all your attention on the chanting.

If you have spoken negatively of someone, you can

---

1 For full instructions of the Divine Light Invocation, see Swami Sivananda Radha, *The Divine Light Invocation,* 3rd ed. (Spokane, WA, USA: Timeless Books, 1990).

undo the negativity by quickly chanting a Mantra and surrounding the person with Light and with the power of the
Mantra. Ask that your weakness not affect the person and
ask to be forgiven. As you become more aware in the moment, you can withdraw what you have said by saying to
those who have heard it, "Please forget I said that. It is
only a one-sided view."

You can also use Mantra to help people you don't
know. When you hear a fire or ambulance siren, for example, say "*Om Namah Sivaya.* Somebody is in need. Let
there be help." If you see pictures in magazines or on television of people killed or injured in war zones, put them
in the Light with Mantra.

When you chant for others, be sure that you are act-
ing out of compassion and not just sympathy. Be aware of
any desire to influence the outcome or any strong emotional response. You must keep your own will out of the
way, surrendering to the power of the Mantra.

What takes place when we chant a Mantra? We attract spiritual power and we offer ourselves as a channel
for this power, that it may pass through us to the sick or
injured person and do whatever is necessary. We must not
demand healing, nor tell God how, when, or how quickly
to accomplish it. We do not know what karma has to be
paid off, or what lessons have to be learned. Healing is not
a hit-or-miss affair, even though to human perception it
may seem so.

Most spiritual healers find, for a variety of reasons,
that not everyone benefits. Sometimes a person who appears
to be a disbeliever is healed while a believer is not. This may
be because the subconscious convictions of these people
are exactly opposite to what they proclaim. The receptivity of the person to be healed is an important element.

The healer must surrender to God, to the Cosmic healing forces, making sure that no personal opinion is held, no judgment made. Only by invoking all the compassion of which you are capable will you be able to invoke, direct, or apply the healing power of the Mantra.

How does one develop compassion? Observe yourself, practice awareness in order to gain understanding of yourself. Wrong conduct must be discarded, not condemned. When you see and forgive your own failings, you will be ready to forgive the failings of others and have more understanding for those you wish to heal. In the process of healing we meet ourselves. Jesus told us to forgive "seventy times seven." He meant us to forgive always, and not to sit in the judgment seat over ourselves or over others.

When you attempt to heal someone, first invoke all the feeling of compassion possible. Put the sick person at ease, helping that person to accept him- or herself without the feeling of being burdened with sin. Healing will not take place with the attitude of "unworthy sinner." Chant the Mantra, and fill yourself with its vibration, thus attracting the forces of the Mantra and channeling them toward the sick person. If you feel that the vibration flows out from the tips of the fingers or the palms, you may hold your hands above the person. Or you can mentally open the doors of your heart and let it flow through. With this vibration flows your own love. It is evidence of your willingness to help.

Confidence will come with success, but do not become over-confident and think that healing will always take place. The Mantra can overcome anything if the person recites it or receives it as a paying off of karma, with trust in forgiveness and a readiness to alter the course of his or her life, dedicating it to the service of God. However, even when a healing has come about, the sickness may return with greater force if the person who was healed does not change a selfish or hurtful way of life. Gratitude to the Divine must be shown in charity or selfless service to others.

Record the results of your efforts in order to increase your understanding of the law of healing. When we call up the spiritual forces we attract, through the vibration of a certain sound or a Mantra, one particular aspect of the Divine Light that is suitable for a specific healing, but perhaps not for all. Much will depend on the makeup of the person who is ill. The influence of such a healing ray can be rejected by the one who is expected to receive it. This does not necessarily take place in the conscious mind but may be a subconscious rejection because of the idea of being unworthy, or of being too great a sinner to expect forgiveness. Sometimes healing is expected too quickly and we give up before it can take place. Not all healing can or should be instantaneous.

When we chant a Mantra we definitely change the sick person's state of mind. We can relax the person and gently probe into the depths of the soul or the mind to find out what resistance we may have to deal with. We can try to help lift the person's burdens. Perhaps we can point out that the Divine really can be trusted, that we have many good reasons for this trust.

May all of you who read this become channels of help and healing and goodness to many others. Bless you all.

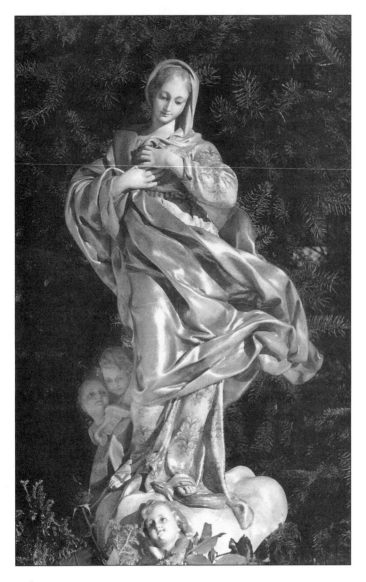

Mary, Queen of Heaven

Chapter Nine

Mantra & Initiation

Arise; awake; approach the teachers and know
the Truth.
The person who is blessed with a teacher knows
the Highest.
He whose devotion to the Lord is great
And who has as much devotion to the Guru as
to the Lord,
Unto him, that high-souled one,
The meanings of the sacred texts stand revealed.

—Quoted from the Upanishads

 All sacred texts and spiritual masters emphasize the need for a teacher on the spiritual path. When you think you have found your Guru, take time to examine yourself and your motives. Do not desire initiation unless you have made up your mind that you want to accept the Teachings and that you will listen and obey. Put aside all worry that you might become dependent on your teacher. A true Guru will lead you to the discovery of the Guru within—your own Higher Self.

Make no demands as to how your Guru should be and how you should be taught. You cannot have a Guru on your own terms. Pray to the Divine that you will be led to a true Guru. Make a bargain with God: ask that the teacher who is your Guru by divine appointment will either say something special to you or greet you in a certain manner, giving you a particular present—a leaf or a flower or a book, whatever you decide. But once you make a promise to God that you will accept the individual who comes to you with that special sign, you must keep your end of the bargain. Don't waste your time Guru-shopping. The teacher will come when the student is ready.

No true teacher will ever ask you to do something that goes against your conscience. It is your responsibility, however, to be clear about your own ideals and principles. When your choice has been made, if you feel that your Guru acts in a way that is not in accordance with your perceptions of spirituality and that you may have made a mistake, remember that the error may be in your perception. Say to the Divine, "I am confused. Is my time with this teacher over? Should I look for another Guru?" Ask for a sign, then wait. If no sign comes, stay with the teacher you have, until the sign you have asked for is given.

Only one who has practiced intensively and has received the power of the Mantra can initiate. Otherwise there is nothing to pass on to the student, in the same way that a father can bequeath to a child only what he himself has already acquired.

A true initiation into a Mantra is like a spiritual marriage between Guru and disciple. It cannot be dissolved by the breaking up of the human relationship; it is only delayed and must be taken up and continued in another life, until the disciple has achieved Self-Realization. The Guru makes a commitment to stay with the disciple through stubbornness, resistance, and avoidance of duty until Self-Realization is achieved. Guru and disciple are always linked through the power of the Mantra. There is an obligation on both sides: the one who initiates accepts responsibility for the disciple, and the initiate must be ready to accept the guidance and authority of the Guru and feel that it is right to take the initiation. According to Swami Sivananda, although it is very difficult to find a teacher who will sincerely look after the interest of the pupil, it is also extremely difficult to find a disciple who will sincerely act according to the instructions of the Guru. His advice to aspirants is to equip themselves with the qualifications of sincerity, humility, and devotion before approaching a Guru, and then not to use reason too much in the selection. For both parties the relationship is an intense one and, because of its duration and importance, must be cherished.

Before the initiation both student and teacher must examine their relationship to see if there is anything that could cause friction between them. These problems should be worked out first. Indeed the student should never accept an initiation until his or her worst weaknesses have been overcome. As Swami Sivananda has said, "The reason for the early downfall of the majority of aspirants is that they imagine themselves to be qualified to adopt the highest form of yoga at the beginning. The qualified aspirant will be humble enough to approach a Guru, surrender himself to the Guru and serve, and learn from him."

As an example of the inflated ideas some aspirants have of their qualifications, one student believed that he could be a teacher because he already felt like one and resented that others did not see him that way. He thought that his saintliness and greatness as a Guru were being purposely retarded by God in order to maintain his interest in helping and guiding others. This is a perverted way of thinking and is an escape from possible criticism for not having the development necessary to be a Guru. Such misconceptions may arise from observing situations in which the Guru may purposely joke or even pretend to be slow or stupid, in order to diminish the fear of some devotees. Or some may naturally, like Swami Purushottamananda, be very childlike, able to take great joy in simple things and find humor in situations that would be unnoticed by others. The awe of the devotee is a hindrance for both Guru and disciple.

In the initiation, or *diksha,* the Guru transmits to the student something of the power of the Mantra. Gurudev Sivananda says, "Initiation gives spiritual knowledge and destroys sin. As one lamp is lit at the flame of another, so the divine Sakti within Mantra is communicated from Guru to disciple." This may be similar to a mild electric shock; it can also be experienced as ecstatic joy, like walking on clouds, lasting for several hours or even a few days. There can be various effects. The power of the Mantra becomes greater after the initiation and will become more perceptible to the disciple, increasing his or her sensitivity. The Mantra then becomes a self-generating force, propelling the disciple into union with the power of the Mantra. The effect on the recipient is dependent on the quality of love and the depth of sincerity with which the power of the Mantra is transmitted.

There is an enormous responsibility in taking initiation. Because the power of the Mantra is neutral, what you do with it can be a blessing to yourself and others, or you can cause great harm.

When you first receive initiation, as in a marriage, there's infatuation and attraction, but human life has its cycles and this period lasts only a couple of years. Then the romance is over. However, you must never break your commitment to your Mantra. Sometimes you will do your practice from a sense of duty, sometimes from love. At some time, you may experience spiritual dryness. This should be understood as a necessary rest period and no foolish decisions should be made about your spiritual future during this time.

When you have received an initiation, there is a commitment to be frank and open with the Guru about the actions and plans of your life. By accepting initiation, you give the Guru the right to intervene in your affairs. The Guru may say no to a proposed marriage or career change, or may ask you to undertake work that is not familiar, or move to a different city. In this relationship, the initiate has someone who cares and who will give advice in an objective manner. Many pitfalls and much pain are thereby avoided. But if this intention of a free exchange dies in the initial stages, it is an obvious signal to both parties that the relationship should be reassessed. There might have been, on the part of the initiate, false hopes of gaining powers or having exciting experiences. If this is the case, the sincerity of the decision must be questioned. Either the full meaning of initiation should be applied, or the relationship dissolved.

Karma will not take effect when there is agreement between parting individuals, assuring that there is no disappointment or pain to either partner. This applies to ordinary marriage and we can therefore reasonably expect that it also applies, to some degree, to the mystical marriage of Mantra initiation.

A one-sided relationship is not really a relationship. There is no better way of describing the purpose and effectiveness of Mantra initiation than in the words of the

Parable of the Sower (Matthew XIII) in which Jesus speaks of the seeds (of Mantra or power) which fall along the path to be devoured by birds, or on rocky ground where the roots wither away, or among thorns where they are choked, and the ones which fall on fertile ground where they grow and bring forth a good harvest.

There are many misconceptions surrounding the idea of initiation. Mantra initiation can take many forms. In India it may be given to children by their father or mother. This took place, for instance, in the life of Papa Ramdas, the renowned saint of Southern India. In these situations the parent is of high spiritual caliber and guides the children's steps with the aim of helping them find the same state of realization. This means that the home life is a highly spiritual one, with study of scriptures, recitation of sacred texts, and invocation of Mantra, as part of daily living. The effect of such early training is deep and lasting. The parent who initiates a child does not have the goal of *sanyas* in mind. (Papa Ramdas was not a *sanyasin.*) It is a blessing for the child and a different kind of Mantra is used.

Mantra initiation may also be given by a compassionate Guru to help an individual, not always on the basis of the recognition of great spiritual potential, but rather on that of need. There may be karmic conditions which are difficult to deal with, and which would make a favorable birth in another lifetime questionable. One of the young fellows in Sivananda Ashram had a record for theft. When I became aware that he had been initiated by Swami Sivananda, I felt that this had been unwise and was puzzled how a Guru could have exercised so little caution. When I asked him why he would initiate such a person, his answer was that by accepting the individual and giving him an initiation he was helping that person to obtain better conditions in another life, and also to give support in the present struggle to overcome weaknesses.

In order for this effort of the Guru to be worthwhile such a disciple would have to possess true humility and a sense of gratitude. Unfortunately, this gratitude may be only temporarily expressed, soon to disappear as if in quicksand. It is clear that, regardless of what the problems are, the Divine will always extend help and it is very foolish to allow pride to stand in the way of accepting and appreciating such a precious gift.

Sometimes a Guru will give "initiation" to a hundred or more people in a special ceremony. Swami Sivananda said this is like putting out a call for the few who can receive the message, who may then come to receive full initiation.

If a Mantra has been received in a dream, usually enough of it is experienced in the dream state to allow the aspirant to recognize the Guru. However, it is entirely at the discretion of the Guru whether or not an initiation will be given. There is no obligation for the Guru to give a Mantra initiation in such cases. Nor is there an obligation just because of contact with a devotee for a number of years, even through living together in the ashram of the Guru. Mantra initiation is not any kind of automatic promotion.

Sometimes Guru and disciple will meet again because of the promise of the Mantra. The disciple will also return when the Guru incarnates to help with the divine work, to repay the time and effort that was spent with the disciple in previous lives. Before his death Ramakrishna indicated when and where he would come back. Those around him asked him jokingly how they would know him and he said that he would carry a hookah! One disciple remarked it would not matter to him because he was not going to re-turn. Ramakrishna replied, "Oh, yes, you will. When the lotus flowers it brings along for its completion all the leaves, buds, and flowers on the stem." This illustrates the respon-sibility that also rests with the disciple, and makes it more clear why the Guru must be informed of actions that may be contrary to the furthering of the work.

The accusation is sometimes made that Gurus dangle initiations before aspirants. There is some reason for think-ing this because the "stick-and-carrot" method is applied by many parents, and companies dangle promotions be-fore people. A Guru who does this may have in mind the objective of collecting many initiates for emotional or eco-nomic purposes, although I have not personally encoun-tered this. If such a suspicion is in the heart of the devotee, the wisest thing would be not to seek initiation from that Guru. As in anything which involves human beings, there will always be good and bad Gurus. The human mind is capable of exploiting anything—the wars which have been fought in the name of various religions are proof of that.

Women must be careful to seek initiation only from a Guru who can accept women as equals. A male teacher who cannot do this is not truly realized. My own Guru, Swami Sivananda, was not a man who had to fear women, or use them, or diminish them to nothing to protect his sexuality. He would work very late at night, and some-times he would call for me to come to his kutir at two o'clock in the morning. I knew I could always go without the slightest fear.

The commitment that is involved in a Mantra initia-tion is not suitable or possible for everybody, but the ideals which it implies may be pursued just as earnestly by those who are not initiated.

The Mantra initiation is an essential first step if the aim is to become a sanyasin. In ashrams it is a general rule that one is initiated by the Guru first into Mantra, followed a few years later by the brahmacharya initiation, and then sanyas. The periods of time between these initiations are meant for intensive study, and for putting into practice what has been learned. The initiation into swamihood gives the right to teach Vedanta and there are different orders of sanyas which have certain distinctions.

Aspirants often ask what would happen to the world if everyone became an initiate, took brahmacharya or sanyas. There is no danger of the world dying out, because there are too many people who want to keep the old games going.

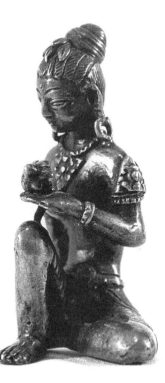

An aspirant making an offering

CHAPTER TEN

Experiences with Mantra

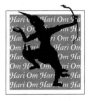 Over the years Mantra has demonstrated its power to me many times. Some of those experiences are included here so that you may understand how Mantra can help a person through the events of life. I have also included some of the experiences of my students to show how a Mantra practice may be approached.

*   *   *

EXPERIENCES WITH OM NAMAH SIVAYA

Once when I was in Montreal, I visited a couple who wanted to have a little satsang, a little prayerful get-to-gether. Suddenly, when we were chanting, the doorbell began ringing fiercely, as if there were a fire. The couple were very alarmed and I, too, knew that something was not right, so I started covering the door with a curtain of Light and reciting *Om Namah Sivaya.*

When the lady of the house opened the door, there was a big fellow standing there, obviously drunk. He said, "Oh, you are having a party. I'll go back to the car and get another bottle." He already had two bottles of whisky in his hands, but he went away, and he didn't come back. The power of the Mantra had done its work. This conveyed to me that Mantra definitely has power.

Another time, when I was traveling—I had many travels because I never refused an invitation, no matter how unpleasant it might be—I accepted an invitation to a group of spiritualists. I was served tea, while the husband told me that his wife was a psychic and could invoke anybody I might want to talk to. I sipped my tea very slowly and with every sip, I repeated silently, "*Om Namah Sivaya,*" with all the power of concentration on the Mantra I could muster.

He asked me if I wanted to summon Shakespeare or one of the great spiritual masters. I said I didn't know of anyone I would want to summon so I would leave it to her.

The woman sat in a corner enclosed in curtains, in a comfortable chair, with a light over her head. She tried, but nobody came. The husband thought perhaps his wife was not in the right mood, so he played me some tapes she had made to show me she could call up anybody. He asked me what I thought about that. I wanted to be very careful not to embarrass him or hurt his feelings, so I said I would have to sleep on it and then I would let him know.

Of course, I did not return to their house, but sometime later the couple came to me in Vancouver. The man was very angry. He said, "You put a spell on my wife. She cannot call any of the masters, not even Shakespeare." He was ready to strike me. Then I said to him, "Did it ever occur to you that your wife could be ready for something much higher?" He became somewhat calm and we talked about gods and goddesses. Finally they left, satisfied.

I have never heard from them since, but there is no question in my mind that when I recited *Om Namah Sivaya* whatever was going to be conjured up couldn't appear because of the protection of the Mantra.

On another occasion, I was driving along the highway with one of the young men from the Ashram. He had a very old car because he gave all his earnings to support the Ashram. Suddenly, he said, "Oh, look. Some car has lost a wheel." I got a very unpleasant feeling in my stomach and I started to say in my mind, "*Om Namah Sivaya, Om Namah Sivaya, Om Namah Sivaya.*" And I heard the young man say, "Oh, my God, that's a wheel from our car!" He was able to stop the car very gently, collect the wheel, and put it back on using some of the bolts from the other wheels. He said to me, "Haven't we been lucky!" I said, "*Om Namah Sivaya* protected us."

AN EXPERIENCE WITH OM TARA

There came a time when I wanted to know more about Tara, but I simply could not get myself to recite her Mantra, which is *Om Tara Tuttare Ture Soha.* So I copied an image of the White Tara from a poster to a piece of cloth and started embroidering it. While I did this, I reflected on the image. Why is her aura red? Isn't red the color of anger? No, not necessarily. Red is also the color of great passion. So I have to approach Tara with great passion. Why does she have seven eyes? As a symbol of all-seeing. The Divine that created the eye doesn't need a physical eye, but for us all-seeing needs to be expressed as physical eyes.

I embroidered every day for a couple of hours for about a year. I didn't recite the Mantra but my mind was focused on Tara. Then one night, I woke myself up with my own voice saying, "I am Tara, I am Radha. I am Radha, I am Tara." This carried on in my waking state for a very long time making it exceedingly difficult to teach classes or to do anything else. There was always this overlay of "I am Radha, I am Tara. I am Tara, I am Radha."

For a long time after this, I wondered how I could substantiate this experience. I know that the mind is a very tricky deceiver and it can make up something even from good desires that isn't necessarily true. Then some students of mine went to India to meet with Tibetan Buddhist nuns to see if they could visit the Ashram. With the permission of the Dalai Lama, whom I had met before, they gave my students a gift for me of one of the twenty-one statues of Tara before which they worshipped daily. My student took a picture of the shelf of Taras showing the empty spot from which it was taken. This Tara is now at the Ashram.

We were also given winter clothes for Tara. They are put on when the cold season begins. It's a kind of warm gesture. Tara is a great spiritual power, a dimension of Divine Mother, and cannot really be touched, but it is very satisfying on a human level to take care of her image and protect it from the cold.

AN EXPERIENCE OF THE KILAKA

Once, when I first started the Ashram, I had a very beautiful experience of the power of the kilaka. There was much work to be done and the young fellows who were at the Ashram then did not always sympathize with my desire to be alone for spiritual practice, or my wish to do spiritual practice rather than help with the painting or the carpentry. One day I was sitting in the garden with my mala, thinking about all the opposition, and I thought, "Perhaps this is not the right time for me to do spiritual practice; I should perhaps wait until I am older and there are more young people here to do the physical work." So I opened my eyes and bent over to pick up my mala.

When I looked up I was amazed to see a circle of people sitting around me. They were all reciting Mantras, moving their beads, moving their lips, looking at me, smiling, and nodding encouragement. I knew then that I had contacted other souls who had gone through the same thing and who were saying, "Come on, stick it out, carry on, we are sitting here with you." This vision gave me the impetus to carry on, and I often had the feeling that other help was given to me.

The struggle to know where my first duty was, to the physical work of the Ashram or to my own spiritual practice, is similar to the conflict which may occur within the family setting. This experience was the answer to the intense conflict within myself over this problem.

EXPERIENCING THE MEANING OF MANTRA

In India, Mantras are often given with no explanation of their meaning, but if they are chanted with perseverence and sincerity, their meaning can become known. Swami Sivananda told me of a young Austrian man who came to see him because his own Guru had died without telling him the meaning of the Mantra he had been initiated into. Swami Sivananda said to him, "You practice the Mantra and write down what you experience until a clear picture emerges." When the young man went back to Austria, he had an experience of his Mantra with Lord Krishna, but he wondered if it was only something his mind had conjured up to satisfy his curiosity. So he asked one of his students to recite the Mantra and to report to him as soon as she had some experience. After six weeks she came back and said she had nothing special to say except that she liked the flute music she heard after reciting the Mantra. He was astounded, and now knew that his Mantra was dedicated to Lord Krishna.

He decided to experiment further. He gave another of his students the last words of Jesus on the cross. After some time, she said to him that she felt compelled to lie on her bed with her arms outstretched. This caused him to become quite alarmed and made him realize that Mantras have much more power than he had recognized.

EXPERIENCES OF MANTRA PRACTICE

I asked a few of my students to provide brief accounts of some of the experiences they have had with their Mantra practices, both at the beginning and over the years. Their experiences may help you in establishing and maintaining your own practice, and show you how very individual is each person's relationship with the Mantra.

Douglas

Chanting appealed to me right from the beginning. During the first yoga workshop I ever attended, I was enthralled, transported even, by the chanting. The words and melodies took hold and stayed with me. Singing was freeing and the words, focused on the Most High, were uplifting.

In grade school, I was one of several students asked to sit down and stop singing. This led to an inhibition about even trying to sing. Mantra chanting helped to change that, as well as changing my voice. Practice and repetition have helped my voice and my hearing. As I hear the subtleties of sound more clearly, I can vocalize them better, and so I *can* sing, even if I never join a choir.

For me to maintain a practice, it is important to set a time of day and a length of time that I will chant. It is also important to set a period—a month, say, or forty days. Doing the practice, whether I feel like it or not, has helped me get over a personality aspect that wants to do what *he* prefers. The freedom from this aspect is wonderful in itself, and persisting in the face of the opposing internal voices has led to some of the most wonderful feelings of connectedness with the Mantra.

I have to beware of my ambition in Mantra practice, for I can fall into a cycle of elation when I am meeting it and depression when I can't meet it. And I have had to go beyond the attitude that if I don't chant for two hours, it doesn't count. My practice goes best when I start small and build on it. I can achieve what I set out to do then, and can build from there by lengthening the practice, or extending the number of weeks or months, or making other changes. I turn to a more intensive, lengthy practice when I experience my emotions getting the better of me. This helps channel and refine the energy. Thus emotion is transformed into devotion.

Mantra has grown to become more and more a part of my life, like brushing my teeth—spiritual hygiene—rather than just an added something I have to do. As part of my thought pattern, it becomes a self-generating force, an automatic reflex that moves my thoughts to the Mantra in times of need, in quiet times, or during work.

Katherine

When I first learned about Mantra, I wanted to know very quickly if there was anything to it before I devoted a great deal of time to it. After the workshop in which I was introduced to Mantra, I chanted aloud for three hours. The day after that, I had to return to my teaching job, and I found that there was indeed something to Mantra. For the next two days, I felt as if I had no skin—as if all my protective mechanisms, good and bad, had been stripped away, exposing my raw nerves. They were two excruciating days, but they convinced me that I was in possession of a powerful tool. I learned that fifteen minutes to begin with is enough, and that the nervous system becomes strengthened through short and regular periods of practice.

I have now been chanting Mantra for many years. It has helped me to dispose of much negativity and to break through the grip of powerful emotions. At times I have sat and chanted for as long as two weeks through an overwhelming but unfocused resentment which I cannot avoid no matter how hard I try. I have learned that this is an expression of subconscious material that the Mantra is bringing up and that if I continue to chant, however difficult, I will become free of it and be able to move on.

Over the years, Mantra practice has been the way I have developed a concept of the Most High, and it has helped me to develop a very personal relationship with the Divine in the form of Divine Mother. I feel that it serves, as Swami Radha says, as a lens for focusing my attention, and at times as a lens for focusing the power of Mantra around me.

Sandra

I feel really blessed to have the gift of Mantra in my life. I was introduced to the chanting of Mantra during a yoga class I attended about eleven years ago. I soon became aware of its calming and elevating effects on my mind.

Within a short time after that, I had to face the possibility of death by cancer. That brought home to me that I did not really know the purpose of my life and here I was presented with losing it. When faced with the possibility of my own death, the rational part of my mind, on which I had always depended, had little to offer. During that very difficult period I made a commitment to make the very best of what life remained for me and to give back to life by supporting Swami Radha's work. My yoga teacher came to chant Mantra with me every day for six weeks. Eventually I recovered. The experience gave me a deep connection with the Mantra and more clarity about the purpose of my life.

I went back to work and soon became involved in the busy and sometimes exhausting demands of my profession. I often had little time or energy to give to Mantra, but I gave what I had. Every day, I would settle myself into a soft, comfortable place on my couch and chant for twenty minutes. To my demanding rational mind, this was not what a Mantra practice ought to be. It was too short; it was too comfortable; and my rational mind did not see how this practice could ever produce the kind of results it wanted. But all I had to offer at that time were my sincerity and faith.

Then I was given a dream of a gong being struck in the center, producing a lovely sound, while a group of people sang "Heart of my heart." To me that dream said my offering was accepted and that somehow through the Mantra I was making a connection with the Divine within through my own spiritual heart. Life took on a different meaning as I realized that it's the Divine that is life, not the body and not the mind.

Janice

I have had a dialogue with Mantra from the first time I heard it in a ten-day yoga workshop. During that workshop, *Om Namah Sivaya* persistently goaded me to look back at my life and investigate it. Now, several years later, this Mantra continues to speak to me, continues to goad me to tap into further truths about my concepts of who I am and what I can do.

After many months of practice, one winter morning while I was chanting it seemed that a silver lining of Mantra formed in the lining of my belly. It is still there, having healed and toughened me up to emotional reactions, both my own and those of others.

It is important to me to continue to feed myself the Mantra, to be nourished by its sound and vibration, never to lose the connection to the source of strength and clarity within. An image that often comes to my mind in connection with Mantra chanting is that of an oil rig, like those set on the prairies, ever deepening and spreading, ever bringing up the rich, dark oil from the depths of my world and beyond.

Mantra is my connection to the Teachings, to the Guru, and to my Higher Self. A friend indeed. I am deeply grateful for this practical and portable treasure.

John

I first experienced Mantra in a Hatha Yoga class in which I was told it would help me perform physically challenging asanas. I discovered that it did. Then, during a ten-day intensive, I experienced the self-generating effect of Mantra as a result of prolonged and constant group chanting. But neither of these experiences helped me to understand what Mantra was.

Some years later in a weekend Mantra workshop, I encountered a different approach brought by a teacher from Yasodhara Ashram. I went, not knowing what to expect. The first session didn't make a lot of sense to me, but I was drawn to chanting and was willing to try. We spent the whole of the next day chanting and writing Mantra. At the end of that day I was ready to quit. However, skeptical as I was, I came back for the final day. At the end, I was calmer, and relieved it was over! It wasn't until the day after the workshop ended, during a business trip to another city, that I started to experience something truly different. I remember most vividly the deep, inner warm sense of assurance. This was the beginning.

Over the last decade and a half, I have learned to use Mantra as a means of leveling emotions and refocusing mentally. Sometimes my practice has been rich and obviously helpful; other times it has seemed dry and empty. There have been deep emotional releases, and through it all I have found another dimension of myself, something that is there everyday, wherever I am.

The scope of this began to reveal itself during a three-month period of seclusion which included an extended Mantra practice of four hours a day—two hours before dawn, one hour before noon, and another after noon. I found the pivotal role Mantra plays in doing in-depth work. I discovered also that there are limits. When I decided to extend the practice to five hours a day, my dreams let me know in no uncertain terms that this was hazardous and unhelpful. Like any tool, Mantra can be used or abused, I found.

Aileen

One of the biggest bridges I needed to cross in my Mantra practice was the one of going from how I thought I *should* do it to finding out what the Mantra means to me and getting involved with it.

The "shoulds" centered around the technicalities of the practice, such as having a straight spine and sitting still. Getting involved with the Mantra changed that around entirely. To be involved meant to open my heart. To act from a "should" meant to operate from my rational mind and to shut down my feelings.

The implications of changing that focus are not immediately apparent, yet in essence the change required changing how I approached my life in general. The obstacle appeared in the Mantra practice, but this way of operating from "shoulds" was happening in many areas of my daily life. Once I began to look, I saw that this right/wrong, good/bad dynamic permeated my mind. Because of the Mantra's effect on the mind—its ability to elevate it out of that literal, limited place—I could see very clearly that something had to change in how I approached my life before I would be able to take the next step on the spiritual path.

Making these changes has been a fluid process as I get more involved with the Mantra and at the same time put the change into daily life by getting truly involved with whatever I am doing. It has meant that I have had to learn to be receptive in both areas of my life, as the one greatly affects the other.

Jay

Initially, chanting Mantra was a very positive experience for me, at times even exhilarating. But my original enthusiasm and wave of early experiences didn't last and it was some time before I could get beyond the obstacles that prevented a deeper, more substantial experience. The early experiences, however, gave a hint of the potential that rested within the sacred syllables, and that indication was strong enough to encourage me to continue the chanting.

In time, I began to see that the obstacles to a deepening practice were creations of my strong intellect. Pride of intellect was the force that refused to open the door to the kind of experience which intellect had already conceptualized as irrational and therefore untrustworthy. Intellectual pride sustains the belief that intellect is superior to the subjective, irrational mind. There was, of course, a lot of support for this position in my western education and socialization process.

But hanging onto my position did not resolve the mental/emotional conflicts that emerged out of my efforts to sustain a practice. I had to learn that the source of the conflict was my fear that intellect would lose control of how I used my mind. The fact that a strong emotion—namely, fear—was controlling my mind eventually showed me I was not using intellect well. I was not using the intellectual power of logic and reason to assess properly and put into language what was happening in my mind during my efforts. The difficulty I went through (and this may be familiar to many men) was created by my not accepting the fact, made evident in the practice itself, that true knowledge—knowledge of the Self—is contained in a side of mind which draws on a very different kind of intelligence.

When I understood, and had some experience of the depth of my mind accessed through chanting, I realized that what I formerly called knowledge was merely information. Chanting Mantra took me over the bridge into a territory of my mind characterized by images, and sometimes by very old memories, which frequently led to powerful emotions and strong feelings. And yet always my chanting would end with a deep sense of peace and well-being, I think because I intentionally directed my chanting toward an image of the Divine—the Radha aspect—to awaken once again the intuitive, devotional part of my nature—the realm of finer feelings and greater sensibility. The intellect cannot give that experience by itself.

I have also found that if the intent of a Mantra practice is to make communion with the Divine, that intention becomes a protection in itself and the length of time for such practice is not as important as the sincerity of effort. In other words, the real matter of importance is: Can I bring all my attention, concentration, and willingness to the chanting even if it is just for a few minutes, and can I invoke enough humility to counter intellectual pride by making the practice an offering? I found I could if I listened intently to the sound created by my voice and breath. Listening calmed the monkey-mind and gave me a way into the heart of the Mantra. By directing my will to listen, I experienced a little of the essence of the Mantra and was able to form a relationship with it that is without fear.

Anne

I have found in my Mantra practice that I need to be involved in other ways than voice alone. It is ritual that provides the basis for my worship. Ritual involves me in the space in which I chant as I set up the altar with its images. It is important to me to arrange flowers, choosing only the best ones for the altar and removing wilting ones; to dust the altar table; to light the candles; to arrange the space so that it is inviting for me and the Divine.

The invitation to the Divine comes from the wonderful fragrance and beauty of the flowers, and from the care and attention I give to the altar. Everything glistens. There is a steadiness that comes from my involvement with the flowers which begins with the choosing of which flowers to grow, tending them, picking them, arranging them on the altar, fragrant and beautiful, and finally removing them to replace them with fresh ones, in a continuing cycle.

At one time I had an image of Tara on the altar. In front of her were seven brass bowls which I would fill with water each morning and each evening empty. As I filled and emptied the bowls, I repeated my own Mantra or the Divine Mother Mantra. This ritual became very meaningful to me because it made my commitment to the Divine visible. If I had not kept my commitment, the water bowls would be empty, quickly reminding me of what I needed to do. Making this gesture before I started chanting also helped to draw me into the Mantra practice. I had a little shawl I would wrap around Tara each night allowing her a private space to rest, then I would wake her up by unwrapping her in the morning Light. I would speak to her, asking for guidance and help, and wait in silence for the part of me which responds when I listen intently within or to the messages from around me. In the chanting of the Mantra, I would use my voice to convey intent and willingness, my wanting, desiring, and longing to be with her. I would ask myself each morning or evening: Are the water bowls full or empty? Is the shawl around her or not? Are the flowers fresh and fragrant? Is my voice clear with my intention? Can I hear her in the silence?

The more involved I am in a ritual, the stronger my commitment becomes to the worship and the richer my practice is.

Carol

I began practicing Mantra as a way to control anger. I had a real problem with it and was directing it toward my husband most of the time. Swami Radha impressed upon me how important it was to deal with this, saying that one outburst of anger used up three years of spiritual practice. This was very difficult because the anger seemed to be beyond my control. I would make all sorts of plans and deals with myself not to react with anger, but all my good intentions were to no avail. The words and emotions were out before I realized what I was doing.

It was my husband who encouraged me to take the problem to the Mantra. I set up a thirty-minute practice for forty days. I chose the *Hari Om* Mantra because of its connection with healing. I prayed that the Divine would help me with making a change and I began the practice. At first I felt comforted by the chanting but there was no change in my behavior. As the days went by, however, I began to feel happier, a little more contented. Then about twenty days into the practice I became aware of a subtle shift or change in me. The anger began to subside of its own accord. I was thrilled and wondered if this would continue. By the end of the forty days I knew that a deep and lasting change had been made. I could feel it and my responses showed it. This experience gave me an understanding of the word "transformation." The anger, or the energy from it, had been transformed into an evenness of temper and compassionate feelings.

I realize now that I had initially been using will-power to try to change and it didn't work. Where the will was really needed was in setting the course of the practice and from there the Mantra could—and did—do the work.

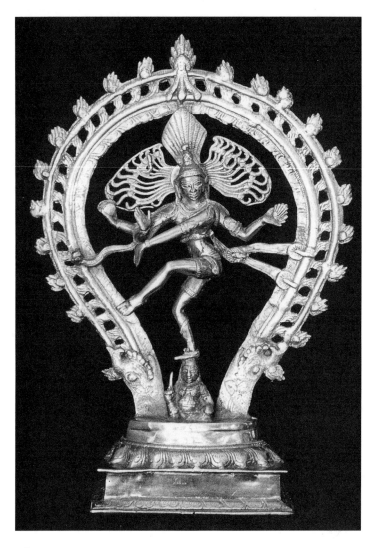

Siva dancing in a ring of fire

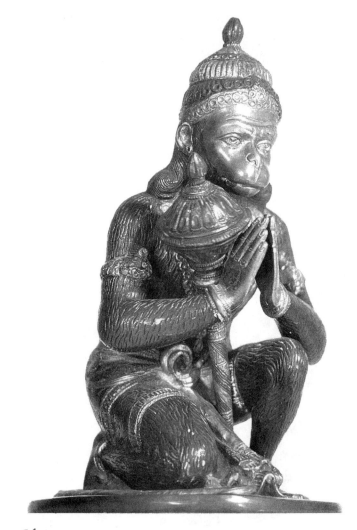

Hanuman, loyal friend to Rama

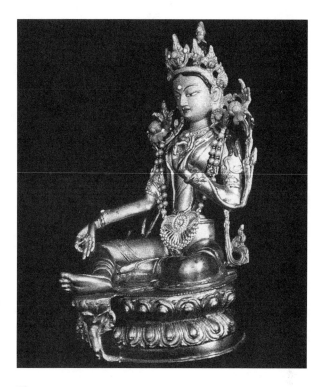

Tara (a gift from the Ganden Choeling Nunnery)

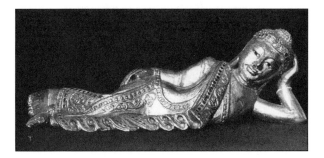

Reclining Buddha

CHAPTER ELEVEN

Mantra in Your Life

 Whatever you achieve through your Mantra practice becomes knowledge which is indestructible. You may lose your life, but the knowledge remains and will reappear in another lifetime. Its purity depends upon how pure a channel you have made of yourself, to what extent you have put your ego aside. Feed your mind the finest food, as you feed your body the most healthful food. Bring quality into your life, refine your senses so that you may become more receptive to the Most High. Do not seek to acquire powers. Whatever the Divine is giving you as a gift or as a signpost that you are on the right path, do not seek to increase that power for some personal end. Do not seek to have power over others. Be grateful and give thanks to the Gurus who have gone before you, because they have opened and prepared the way.

When you feel critical of yourself or others, counteract this by chanting a Mantra in your mind. Let the Mantra truly take over and purify the mind and you will see the blessings that come to you. That effort may sometimes seem beyond your capabilities. When you feel that way, resort to prayer and ask for help. It is an act of humility to realize that you cannot do it all by yourself. Those who have achieved Cosmic Consciousness before you will respond and bring you, too, close to that state.

Do not hesitate to cry at the feet of the Divine about your unworthiness because the Divine will make you worthy. If you have received a Mantra initiation there must be some worthiness, but it is your responsibility and obligation to demonstrate it. God and Guru work with you but they do not carry you, they do not work for you. Yoga is the path of revelation and liberation. You have to take the first step.

When you chant the name of God the work you do becomes easier, more joyful; it is no longer a distasteful duty because the Mantra will be continuously in the back of the mind, bringing the attention back to God and to the thought that God is working through your mind and hands.

By chanting or reciting, aloud or silently, you carry the force, the power of the Mantra and this power will be a blessing wherever you go. But remember that it is from the Mantra, not your personality, that the blessing comes. By mentally repeating your Mantra when others come to you with their problems, you prevent the thinking process from obstructing intuition. However, do not think that you always have to have the answer. You may not be the channel for this person, or your silence may be their best lesson at this point.

For people living an ordinary life in the world, all

the practice and work in self-development will build a foundation for the time when they can pursue a more intense search for higher values and the spiritual goal. It is good for everyone to chant a Mantra while engaged in such routine tasks as washing dishes, scrubbing floors, or cutting the grass, because in these the mind is left relatively free and much energy can be wasted in allowing it to drift. These tasks provide an opportunity for self-purification.

At the end of the day do not watch the news or have an argument, because at this most susceptible time you will take the anger and violence into your dreams. Instead take a positive message with you when you go to sleep by playing a Mantra tape or chanting your Mantra. You can train yourself to keep the Mantra with you all night during sleep. As you switch off the light, think that you are symbolically switching off all daily activity, then lie quietly and recite your Mantra. Soon the Mantra will take over because at this time, when the power of suggestion is at its strongest, the energy of the Mantra is most active.

Learn to keep the Mantra going in your mind at all times. Use the various forms of Japa—Likhita, Vaikhari, Upamsu, Manasika—alternating them with chanting, depending on the occasion, or to give your busy mind the variety it wants. It does not matter if others think you strange to be writing or whispering to yourself. Be God's fool—the Pearl of Great Price is worth the price. Practice until you get results. Do not give up!

Salutations and Gratitude to All the Gurus
Who Have Prepared the Way.

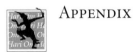 Appendix

From the Writings of Swami Sivananda of Rishikesh, India

The following are excerpts from various writings of Swami Sivananda Saraswati. He was my great Guru, who instructed me to put the yogic teachings into a form that could be understood by the Western mind. His work has been an inspiration to me all my life. I include some of his writings here so that others may experience something of his greatness and enthusiasm, and as an expression of gratitude for all that he gave me.

A DISCIPLE—FAITH CAN WORK MIRACLES

A great Guru who lived in a temple on the bank of a broad river and had many hundreds of disciples all over, once summoned his disciples, saying that he wanted to see them before his death, which was to take place soon. The most favourite disciples of the great Guru, who always lived with him, grew anxious and kept themselves close to him day and night. For they thought that he might disclose to them at last the secret which made him so great, and all of them fearing lest they should miss the great opportunity, watchfully awaited the moment when the secret would be revealed. For, though their Guru taught them many sacred Mantras, they acquired no powers and hence thought that the Guru still kept to himself the method which made him great. Disciples from everywhere arrived every hour and awaited with great expectation.

Now a humble disciple who lived far away on the opposite side of the river also came. But the river which was in high flood was too turbulent even to allow boats to pass. However, the humble disciple must not wait, as in the meanwhile the Guru may pass away. He should not tarry; but what was to be done? He knew that the Mantra which his Guru taught was all-powerful and capable of doing anything. Such was his faith. So, chanting the Mantra with faith and devotion he walked over the river. All the disciples who saw this were surprised at his powers. And recognising him as the one who came long ago to their Guru and stayed but one day and went away after being taught something by him, all the disciples thought that the Guru had given him the secret. They sternly demanded of their Guru why he deceived them thus, though they served him in every humble manner for many years, and yielded the secret to a stranger who came there for a day, long ago.

The Guru, with a smile, waved them to be calm, and summoning the humble disciple to his presence, ordered him to tell the disciples what he was taught by him long ago. The anxious group of disciples was taken aback with amazement when they heard him utter the name of "Kudu-Kudu" with awe, veneration, and devotion. "Look," said the Guru, "in it he believed, and thought that he got the clue to all. And even so is he rewarded for his faith, concentration and devotion. But you always doubted, thinking that something remained unrevealed still, though I told you Mantras of great powers. This distracted your concentration, and the idea of a great secret was in your mind. You were constantly thinking about the imperfection of the Mantra. This unintentional and unnoticed concentration upon the imperfection made you imperfect."

THE DISCIPLE AND THE TEMPLE

There was once a temple in a small mountain city near a holy river. The temple had a door that closed very firmly—and had no handle. The only way the door could be opened was by chanting the Lord's name. Every few years all the saints and sadhus were invited to come to the temple and take turns at sitting, chanting one of the names of God, before the temple doors. If God accepted their offering, He would Himself open the door.

Now, not far from the city was a cave, in which was living a very famous Mantra singer, and a young man, and they shared their practice time together. They slept the same length of time, ate together and spent their meditation time together. The cave was very small so it was necessary for them to coordinate their activities so as not to disturb one another. And as they both worshipped the same aspect of God there was a harmony between them as perfect as can be among spiritual people.

In accordance with tradition, they went to the temple and the opportunity to chant before the temple doors was given first to the older man. When his turn came, he sat before the door and sang his heart and soul out to God. After two weeks the doors opened with a bang.

So the younger man's turn came and he, too, sat before the temple doors and chanted. A week passed, two weeks, three weeks. According to the tradition no one was refused to sit before the temple door and chant, however long he may spend there. The young man chanted for a month, two months, and as the weeks went by three months passed. Then, suddenly, with a great clap of thunder, the doors of the temple burst open and everyone present was thrown to the ground by the shock.

The young man went home and sat under a tree and wept. He said, "Lord, am I so far away, so very far away from You that it has taken me this long to open the temple doors? What have I done? Please tell me." And the Lord granted His beloved devotee a vision and said, "Put aside all your worries, my child. I was so delighted with your singing that I forgot to open the door."

A REAL GURU

Here are the characteristics of a real Guru. . . . He has full knowledge of the Self and Vedas. He can remove the doubts of aspirants. He has equal vision and a balanced mind. He is free from . . . egoism, anger, lust, greed, . . . and pride. In his presence one gets Santi and elevation of mind.

India, the sacred land of Adwaita philosophy, the land which produced Sri Sankar, Dattatreya, Vam Dev and others who preached oneness of life and unity of consciousness, is full of sectarians now. . . . it is difficult to count the number of sects that are prevailing now in India. . . . Hopeless discord and disharmony reign everywhere. . . . The disciples of one Guru fight with the disciples of another Guru. . . .

Lord Chaitanya, Sri Guru Nanak, Swami Dayananda were all catholic, exalted souls. All their teachings were sublime and universal. They never wanted to establish sects or cults of their own. Had they lived now they would have wept at the actions of their followers. . . .

A spiritual teacher should never establish a sect of his own. Founding a sect means creation of a fighting centre to disturb the peace of the world. . . . He can have an institution with broad, universal principles and doctrines that will not conflict with the principles of others and that can be universally accepted and followed by all.

Some [spiritual teachers] . . . made no Ashrams . . . gave no lectures . . . made no disciples, yet their names were handed down . . . as ideal, spiritual personages. They have created . . . an indelible impression on the minds of people by their exemplary lives. . . . The vibrations of a realized soul do purify the whole world even if he remains in a far-off cave in the Himalayas. . . .

Can a patient gauge the merits of a doctor as soon as he enters the consultation room? Ignorant disciples who have no experience in the spiritual path at once begin to test and examine their Guru. They make hasty conclusions and inferences from external appearances and ways of living. . . . Even though you live with [realised souls] . . . you can hardly understand their hearts and depth of knowledge. Jnana and spiritual experiences are internal states.

A young man with a little training . . . poses [as] a Guru. . . . Ignorant worldly people are deceived. . . . Ladies are very easily duped, easily attracted by sweet music and melody. . . . These Gurus . . . easily influence them . . . make them their tools or instruments. . . exploit them. . . . Open your eyes. . . . Use your reason. . . . Beware of posing Gurus. . . . Some make disciples to get services when they become old.

DEVOTION TO GURU

Guru is Brahman Himself. . . . A word from him is a word from God. Even his presence or company is elevating, inspiring and stirring. . . . Living in his company is spiritual education. . . . He knows the spiritual path. He knows the pitfalls and snares on the way. He gives timely warnings to the students. . . . It is he who overhauls the old, wrong, vicious Samskaras of aspirants, removes the veil of Avidya, all doubts, Moha, fear, etc., awakens the Kundalini and opens the inner eye of intuition.

A thirsty aspirant who has implicit faith in his Guru and who is very eager to imbibe the teachings, can only drink the nectar from him. The student can imbibe from his Guru in proportion to the intensity and degree of his faith in him.

The Guru tests students in various ways. Some students misunderstand him and lose their faith in him. Hence they are not benefitted.

The student and the teacher should live together as father and devoted son, with extreme sincerity and devotion. The aspirant should have an eager receptive attitude to imbibe the teachings of the master. Then only will the aspirant be spiritually benefitted.

In the initial stages, an aspirant will have to face many difficulties and doubts on his path. He must have somebody whom he can approach to get his doubts cleared.

You should be careful in selecting the Guru. Do not be carried away by the belief that somebody is a great Mahatma. . . . You should not change your Guru after choosing one. . . . Live with [the Guru and his disciples] or move among them for some time. . . . If he puts forth a contrary view to the one you hold, listen to it by all means, but do not change your central, basic principle. . . .

It is only the Guru who will find out your defects. The nature of egoism is such that you will not be able to find out your own defects. . . . In the spiritual path you will have to take out your bones, crush them into powder and extract oil from it and burn the wick with this oil for several years. Only then, will God appear before you. . . . What is the nature of your goal? It is immortality. To attain this should you not strive hard?

Karma Yoga is very necessary for man's evolution. . . . Ethical perfection can only be got by following the instructions of your Guru and by selfless service. . . . Work is worship for a Karma Yogin. . . . This is the way to annihilate your pride and vanity and false notion of superiority.

Energy is indestructible. What I have said will not go in vain. When a sound is uttered, it is not lost. And those who are in tune with my vibrations will be benefitted by my speech.

GURU AND DISCIPLE

As man is under the influence of beginningless ignorance, he needs the help of a Preceptor to have Self-Realisation. Just as a man cannot see his back, so also he cannot see his own errors.

When you live with your Guru, you must be prepared to do willingly any work assigned by him.

An aspirant who attends on his Guru with great devotion in his personal services, quickly purifies his heart. This is the surest and easiest way for self-purification.

Intense devotion to one's Guru and faithful adherence to his teachings are the most essential qualifications of true discipleship. . . . Gurubhakti draws down the grace of the Preceptor and bestows ultimately illumination and bliss. . . . The grace of the Guru flows towards the disciple if the latter has a true receptive attitude and sincere faith in his Guru.

One's individual ego, preconceived notions, pet ideas and

prejudices and selfish interests should be given up. These stand in the way of carrying out the teachings and instructions of one's Guru. . . . Do total self-surrender to obtain the Guru's Grace. . . . Love of Guru should engender love for the whole universe, because you must see him in all.

The spiritual path is not like writing a thesis for an M.A. It is quite a different line. The help of a teacher is necessary at every moment. Young aspirants become self-sufficient, arrogant, and self-assertive these days. They do not care to carry out the orders of a Guru. . . . They want independence from the very beginning. They apply in an absurd manner, with a perverted intellect, the Neti-Neti Doctrine.

If you cannot get an ideal Guru, you can take even a man who has been treading the path of realisation for some years, who is straightforward and honest, who is selfless, who is free from pride, egoism, who has good character, who has good knowledge of the Sastras.

Beware of pseudo-gurus . . . [who] will exhibit tricks or feats to attract people. . . . Do not be deceived by their sweet talk.

Guru and disciple should be well acquainted with the nature of the other. The student should be able to know thoroughly well the ideas and principles of his Guru and the Guru must be able to detect the mistakes and imperfections in the student. The Guru should be allowed to make a complete study of the aspirant's inner nature. . . . The disciple should lay bare all weakness and shortcomings . . . allow himself to be tested in the crucible of sufferings by his Guru so the Guru may have full confidence in him.

GURU AND INITIATION

It is better if you get your Mantra from your Guru. This has a tremendous effect on the disciple. The Guru imparts his Shakti along with the Mantra. If you cannot get a Guru, you can select any Mantra according to your own liking and taste, and repeat it mentally, daily, with Shraddha and Bhava. This also has a great purification effect. You will attain the realisation of God.

The method of initiation need not . . . be the same for every aspirant. According to the yearning of the aspirant the Lord will arrange his guide suited to the temperament of the Sadhak.

Initiation, inspiration and the attainment of knowledge depend upon the aspirant's personal efforts and his earnestness. The Lord's grace descends on him at the proper time, when his patient and sustained struggle for realisation is no longer necessary.

Some like Yogi Milarepa have to serve their masters arduously for a long time whereas some get the initiation in a flash. It depends upon the spiritual Sadhana and evolution of the Sadhak. Yogi Milarepa underwent a series of struggles during his service of his Guru. He had to perform superhuman acts of heroism and bravery before he was initiated. Sages and Rishis of yore put their students to severe trials before they took them into their confidence. They intuitively knew whether a student was fit for initiation. The neophytes were entrusted with the work of tending the cow, bringing fuel from the forest for the Ashram, washing the clothes of the Guru and other such works which look like menial service in the eyes of the present day Sadhaka. For Sadhaks like Swetaketu, Indra, Satyakama and others every act was an act of Yoga or worship of the Guru. To them nothing was menial. They dedicated everything to their masters with unselfish motive. Therefore, they quickly attained Chitta Shuddi, studied and mastered the Vedas and finally acquired the knowledge of the supreme Self.

Gautama chose four hundred lean weak cows and asked Satyakama Jabala, his disciple, to tend them and instructed him not to return before they became one thousand.

The aspirant, before he desires the grace of the master, should deserve it. The supply of divine grace comes only when there is a real thirst in the aspirant and when he is fit to receive it.

If a Bhakta-saint is approached by an aspirant who wants to tread the path of knowledge, the former may direct the latter to the proper Guru for initiation. . . . But a saint of perfect realisation can give initiation in any path.

It is very difficult to know the particular Yoga by which the Guru reached perfection unless he himself reveals it to the aspirant out of compassion. No Sadhak will be bold enough to put this question to his Guru lest he should be considered impertinent.

Except in cases of advanced Sadhaks, initiation comes after a long and patient service to the preceptor.

The disciple should come in close contact with the Guru during his service and try to imbibe all his good qualities.

If the fault-finding nature is strong in the disciple, he cannot pick up anything from the preceptor and his spiritual progress will be at a standstill.

In the absence of a realised Sad-Guru, senior aspirants who have trodden the spiritual path for a long time, who are above base desires, who have served their preceptors for a long time, and who are Sannyasins also can help a neophyte. . . . If one is not able to find such an advanced aspirant, one can follow the teachings contained in the books written by realised saints . . . keep a photo of such a realised Guru and worship the same with faith and devotion. Gradually the aspirant will receive inspiration. The Guru may appear in a dream and initiate and inspire him at the proper time.

The disciple becomes like his Guru after some time by following his instructions. . . . A disciple is he who follows the instructions of the Guru to the letter and spirit, who propagates the teachings of the Guru to less evolved souls in the path, till the end of his life.

ARE YOU REALLY QUALIFIED ?

The spiritual aspirant must have faith and devotion to Guru and the Lord . . . intense aspiration and dispassion . . . lead a contented life, and possess the three fundamental virtues— Ahimsa, Satyam and Brahmacharya . . . be gentle, humble and noble.

The aspirant has to . . . observe moderation in everything and lead a well-regulated, disciplined life of perfect celibacy and self-restraint . . . discipline the senses . . . possess a loving heart . . . never injure the feelings of others . . . not be jealous.

He has no right to compare his privileges with those of others. If a thing is refused to him he should not aspire for it again. Without the spirit of selfless service and self-denial it is very difficult to progress.

The Sadhak must speak gently, sweetly and truthfully . . . always be cheerful, earnest, vigilant and diligent.

He must possess adaptability, courage, mercy, generosity, tolerance, patience, perseverance and discrimination. He should bear insult and injury, have equanimity, fortitude and forbearance.

His speech must agree with his thought, and his action must agree with his speech.

Even for a single day he should not miss introspection and self-analysis.

He must stick to his ideal and should be ever aware of his goal.

Never despair; be hopeful always. Persist in your practice.

Even in the study of secular science and worldly matters you need the help of a teacher. You cannot understand science, mathematics, algebra, geometry without the aid of a teacher. . . . Is it not much more necessary, then, to have a Guru in transcendental matters, when the aspirant has to walk along the rugged, thorny spiritual path?

Guru's Grace alone will sustain you in the perilous spiritual path which is as sharp as the edge of a razor.

Even Sri Sankara, Lord Krishna, Lord Rama, Sri Ramanuja, and Ekanath, had their Guru.

THE FOUR MEANS

A student who treads the path of Truth must equip himself with the four means of salvation or Sadhana Chatushtaya viz., Viveka, Vairagya, Shad-Sampat and Mumukshatva. . . . These four means are as old as the Vedas or this world itself. Every religion prescribed these four essential requisites for the aspirant. Names only differ.[1]

Let me sound a note of warning here. . . . Vairagya [dispassion] also may come and go if you are careless and mix promiscuously with all sorts of worldly-minded persons. You should develop Vairagya to the maximum degree. The mind is so constituted that it is waiting like a vulture to get back the things once renounced . . . you should take refuge in Viveka [discrimination] and in the impenetrable fortress of wise, dispassionate Mahatmas.

There are different degrees in Vairagya. Supreme dispassion comes when one gets himself established in Brahman. The Vairagya becomes perfectly habitual.

The desire for sensual enjoyment is deep-rooted or ingrained in the minds of all. The Rajasic mind is so framed that it cannot remain even for a single moment without thoughts of enjoyment of some kind or another. People invent various sorts of subtle enjoyments. Modern science has made marvellous contributions towards bringing forth refined ways of enjoyment. Modern civilisation is only another name for sensual enjoyment . . . hotels, cinemas, aeroplanes, radios . . . new dishes, new syrups, new drinks . . . fashion in dress . . . the hair. Even the man who is treading the path of Truth wishes to find lasting and intense sensual enjoyments by means of his Yogic practices. He wants to taste the nectar of immortality . . . hear the music of celestial nymphs . . . These are the subtle temptations. The sincere aspirant will resolutely turn his back from all sorts of refined, subtle, intense forms of enjoyments herein and hereafter.

THE GREATEST FACTOR IN SPIRITUAL REALISATION

A true disciple is concerned only with the Divine Nature of the Guru. The Guru's action as man is not the disciple's concern. . . . Always remember that the nature of a saint is un-

---

1   *Viveka*—discrimination; *vairagya*—dispassion; *shad-sampat*—six-fold virtue bringing about mental control and discipline; *mumukshatva*—intense desire for liberation.

fathomable. . . . Measure not his divine nature with the inadequate yardstick of your ignorance.

He who initiates Mantra is Diksha-Guru or initiatory Guru.

He who teaches the various forms of Sadhana and Yoga is Shiksha Guru or the teaching Guru.

Of these two, he is the supreme Guru from whom the great Mantra of Ishtadevata has been heard and learnt and by him alone Siddhi can be attained.

Competent disciples are never in want of a competent Guru.

The disciple achieves results in proportion to his faith in his Guru.

The possession of a university degree cannot entitle a man to be an examiner of a Guru.

It is the height of impertinence and foolishness on his part, blinded by the vanity of worldly knowledge, to test the spiritual knowledge of the Guru.

The Guru teaches through personal example. Learn it and act wisely.

The day-to-day conduct of the Guru is the living ideal to the disciple who is observant.

The true Guru is like a central power-house. He electrifies his disciples.

Mantra-Diksha is indeed a very rare and unique good fortune. Receive it with the utmost reverence and pure spiritual bhav.

A God-realised Sadguru never dies in the ordinary sense. He is ever present, as he has identified himself with the Immortal Cosmic Being. To sincere disciples, he can appear whenever he wills.

Worship the Guru always. . . . The highest form of worship of Guru is meticulous practice of his teachings and living by his example.

The relation between a Guru and disciple is real, sacred and everlasting.

Learn how to obey. Then only you can command.

Learn how to be a disciple. Then only you can become a Guru.

Listen to all but follow one. Respect all, but adore one. Gather knowledge from all, but adopt the teachings of one Master.

Correct understanding, non-attachment to worldly objects, serenity of mind, restraint of the senses, absence of base passions, faith in the Guru and devotion to God are necessary equipment with which the aspirant has to approach the Guru.

Satsang or association with the Guru is an armour and fortress to guard you against all temptations and unfavourable forces of the material world.

The mission of the saints is to save those lost in ignorance of the path leading to God.

The words of a saint go straight to the heart of hearers and cling there.

Saints do the great work of distillation. They raise the souls to purity, perfection, freedom and union with God.

The ink of a sage or Yogi is more precious than the blood of a martyr. A saint or a sage is a Teacher. He is a healer, harbinger of light, love, peace, strength and solace to the weary and heavy laden heart of humanity.

OUR WEDDING IS INDISSOLUBLE!

"Sorrow not, my child. Sit down. In this world of phenomena such things do happen in the natural course of events. It is nobody's fault. When two minds come together, misunderstandings are natural. Sometimes quarrels do arise. Eventually the love of the heart overcomes all and cements the differences."

"It is not always possible for any two persons, however highly evolved they may be, to be always thinking alike and feeling alike. No two minds can ever agree. This is because each one is guided by one's own peculiar desires and cravings, ambitions and aspirations, and in adjusting our conduct their fulfilment becomes a joyous sacrifice on our part. If we have the spirit of service the very desires and ambitions in the other person would help us manifest our own spirit in a greater and greater measure."

"Inordinate attachment to things often causes an aggravation of disharmony."

"Such is the relationship between a Guru and his disciple . . . for it is on the plane where everything is Eternal. You and I have been together not only in this incarnation, but in so many of our past lives. Our relationship is irrevocable."

A SELF-SACRIFICING DISCIPLE

Sri Gopala received his initiation from his Guru, Swami Santananda, in Benares. The Guru said: "Look here, my dear Gopala; you will attain Moksha by recitation of this Mantra. But do not reveal this Mantra to anybody. If you reveal it, you will go to hell."

Sri Gopala was an aspirant of a very large heart. He at once went to the market and recited the Mantra openly before a large assembly of persons. He spoke plainly: "You all can attain salvation through the recitation of this Mantra. It was given to me by my Brahma Nishta Guru. My guru told me that I would go to hell if I reveal it to other people. I am prepared to go to hell. But I am exceedingly glad to see that you all will attain Salvation."

Swami Santananda was passing along the market road. He heard the candid speech of his large-hearted, sympathetic disciple Sri Gopala. He was highly pleased with his sincere disciple and said: "My dear Gopala, you will also attain Moksha this very second. You are a noble, magnanimous soul. I want disciples of your description." Aspirants should develop Udaratta to a considerable extent. This will induce oneness, unity and cosmic love. It will generate Adwaitic feeling. It paves a long way to the attainment of Moksha.

THE TECHNIQUE OF PERFECTION

Seekers of Truth!

The desire to seek help, to search for light, to look up to higher powers, is inborn in all beings. The incapacity to achieve the ideal of the aspirations that spring from the heart, the anguish which accompanies such incapacity, and the knowledge of the existence of superior powers, obliges individuals to take shelter under those that are endowed with the ability to lift them up to higher levels. The world is a dramatic scene of dependence of beings on others that can fill up what they lack. Love for God means the yearning to reach the highest, to become perfect, and this is not easy for all who wish to be so.

Perfection has its center in the core of the seeker himself and hence the difficulty of knowing the exact technique of realising it, which is God, Self, and all that is best. The key to the door that opens into the realm of truth and perfection does not lie in those who see through the intellect, but those who intuit the reality in integral comprehension, not as an object lying outside, but as rooted in the very meaning of the subject. These are called the seers or the sages, the Brahmanishtas who can communicate the spiritual consciousness even through a glance or a touch or through a single command. They are the Gurus or the Masters who teach the truth to and shower God-consciousness on the mortals. Patanjali Maharishi says that Ishwara himself is the greatest Guru, for he is the most ancient and is omnipresent and, being the seed of omniscience, he is the teacher of all teachers, unsullied by the changes of time. To surrender oneself to God is, therefore, to seek shelter under the origin of knowledge, the source of power, the Lord of creation itself.

Guru is not the human personality. Guru is the Divine Being, the immortal essence that shines through the human person. The perishable body constituted by the physical elements should not be mistaken for the Guru. The real teacher is the one Brahman that manifests itself as and when it likes. Man can learn only from a human and hence God teaches man through a human body. The human body of the Guru is an occasion to worship his universal nature of supreme Light, a nail to hang the shirt on. The human side of the Guru is not what is important, it is the unseen but the only real Atman, the ubiquitous principle that underlies it, that is the true Guru. When we pray to God, we pray not to a body. When one resorts to a Guru, he does not do so to a material form. The dignified substratum of life, light and joy, the grand consciousness that soars above the paltry grandeur of the universe, that is what is to be seen in a

Guru! "Hit it, O Somya," says the Upanishad. That is the target of meditation and the object of devotion, the teacher and the saviour, the support and the goal. Lord Krishna says, "Know me 'in truth'," where he emphasizes the fact that his form, the body, is not to be mistaken for the Eternal. Guru is God and God is Guru, and the Svetaswatara Upanishad says that the truth is revealed to that great-souled one who does not consider God and Guru as two different beings.

The sacred relation of Guru and disciple is a very ancient one. Even from Vedic times we hear of the necessity of the aspirants seeking Brahma-Srotriyas and Brahmanishtas being stressed. "Examining the worthless nature of the action-bound world the wise one should get disgusted with it, for the eternal cannot be reached through action. For the sake of knowing That he should resort to a Guru, well versed in spiritual lore and also established in Brahman-consciousness," says the Mundaka Upanishad. Though the Guru does not actually give anything not already possessed, he becomes the means which digs out the spiritual wealth that is buried under the ignorant mind of the aspirant. Since all experiences in the world are the effects of the interaction of the knower and the known, the spiritual experience too is in a different way the effect, as it were, of the union of subjective endeavour and the object presented before it, be it physical or purely psychical, be it embodied teachers or bodiless mental forms or ideas.

It is from the Guru that the seeker gets the influx of spirituality and divine Bhava. What the aspirant receives, he intensifies and multiplies a thousand-fold through earnest Sadhana. This is the duty of all aspirants. The Guru is the gateway to the transcendental Truth-consciousness, but it is the aspirant that has to enter through it. The Guru is a help but the actual task of practical Sadhana falls on the aspirant himself.

In truth the Guru dwells in your heart. The Guru is ever by your side. You have only to think of him with real Bhava and you will at once feel his spiritual presence without fail. In proportion to the effacement of the lower ego does the Guru manifest in you and appear before you. Therefore be ever ready to receive him and empty yourself of all contents so that he may fill himself in you.

TALKS WITH THE ASPIRANTS

Is a Guru Necessary?

A Guru is absolutely necessary for everyone. In the initial stages an aspirant will have to face many difficulties and doubts in his path. He must have somebody whom he can approach to get his doubts cleared. Even ordinary secular sciences have to be learnt from a teacher. To learn the Science of science, Brahma Vidya or Self-knowledge, the help of a Guru is absolutely essential. It is only the Guru who will find out your defects. The nature of egoism is such that you will not be able to find out your own defects. In the case of a very few exalted souls, their own Self serves as their Guru and guides them from within; but this is due to the fact that they have in their previous births performed intense Sadhana with the help and guidance of Brahma Vidya preceptors.

Only the man who has already been to Badrinath will be able to tell you the road. In the case of the spiritual path it is still more difficult to find your way! The mind will mislead you very often. The Guru will be able to remove pitfalls and obstacles and lead you along the right path. He will tell you: "This road leads you to Moksha; this one leads to bondage."

Some might find their own inner conscience is their Guru. It will guide them aright. They, too, have ascended the steps of the ladder of yoga through service of the Guru and through his instructions in their previous births. Their heart is so pure that doubts do not arise at all in them. They are, so to say, born Siddhas.

Whom shall I choose as my Guru?

He who is able to clear your doubts, he who is sympathetic in your Sadhana, he who does not disturb your beliefs but helps you on from where you are, he in whose very presence you feel spiritually elevated—he is your Guru. Once you choose your Guru, implicitly follow him. God will guide you through the Guru.

Do not use your reason too much in the selection of your Guru. You will fail if you do so. If you fail to get a first-class Guru, try to follow the instructions of the Sadhu who [has been] treading the path for some years, who has purity and other virtuous qualities and who has some knowledge of the scriptures. Just as a student of an intermediate class will be able to teach a student of the Third Form when a Professor with M.A. qualifications is not available . . . this second-class type of Guru will be able to help you.

* * *

It is the duty of saints and elder Sannyasins to protect spiritually thirsting aspirants.

The aspirants of today need not renounce the world and run to the forest in search of a Guru. Some will, no doubt, do so; and they will eventually act as the spiritual guides to the rest of humanity. The vast majority would, however, have to learn at home and practise Yoga in their daily life, to learn and apply the technique of transforming their daily actions into Yoga Sadhana.

The teacher and the seeker should meet half-way. This divine meeting place is a spiritual institution, Ashram or Math.

The worship and adoration of the Guru is the first step to Cosmic Consciousness.

The vision of the Guru will slowly expand. You will, under the wise guidance of the illuminated Guru, gradually perceive that Supreme Principle that resided in your Guru pervades the entire creation. When the inner consciousness expands, there will be nothing to obstruct it, no ego to limit its expansion. You will very soon realise Cosmic Consciousness. This is the Supreme secret of service of Guru, worship of Guru and self-surrender to Guru. First realise your God in your Guru. Then you will realise God in everyone. First serve your Guru selflessly. Then you will be able to serve the entire humanity selflessly. First worship your Guru with sincerity and devotion. Then you will worship the All-pervading Lord. Guru is the gateway to God-realisation.

Guru is the sacred altar at which you can willingly and lovingly sacrifice your ego.

It is the Guru who removes the veil of ignorance. Serve him with Bhakti. Then you will get his Grace. The physical form of the Guru will slowly vanish. You will realise the Atma in and through him. You will see your Guru in all forms, animate and inanimate.

The greatest service that I can do to humanity is training and moulding of aspirants. Every Yoga student, when he is purified and elevated, becomes a centre of spirituality. He will draw to himself through his magnetic aura thousands of baby-souls in spirituality for transformation and regeneration.

If you think that I am worthy enough, you can take me as your Guru.

Realised souls are not rare. Ordinary ignorant-minded persons cannot easily recognise them. Only a few persons who are pure and embody all virtuous qualities can understand realised souls and they only will be benefitted in their company.

Testing a guru is highly difficult. Do not use your intellect here. Have faith. The real aspirant is quite free from such questions and doubts. You will be miraculously helped if you believe in my words.

I am neither a Guru nor a Sat-Guru. I take great delight in serving others.

Fail not to observe the vow of celibacy at any cost.

Every Sannyasi, every Yogic student has some defect or other. It is only a full-blown Yogi or a Jnani who will be absolutely free from evil qualities and defects . . . [such] are rare. . . . Slight friction is bound to come between friends, at times between Sannyasins too. One must excuse the other, must reunite and forget the past. You must have a tendency to grasp only the good in others. . . . Everyone has some virtues. No one is entirely bad. Remember the point well. After some time you will find only good in others. . . .

If you cannot get a suitable Guru, you can select any Mantra according to your inclination and repeat the same with great faith in the power of the Mantra. Any Mantra is powerful. Stick to one and to one form. Do not change.... Aspirants who have no faith in the Mantra, after some practice, jump to another. To avoid this, it is advised to get a Mantra from a Guru. Further the Guru imparts his special power to the disciple through the Mantra at the time of Diksha.

I continuously work, read and write. I never go to hill-stations or sea-side for a holiday, change of work gives rest. Meditation gives abundant rest.

I am a strange mixture of service, devotion, Yoga and wisdom. I am a follower of Sri Sankara. I am a Keval-Adwaita Vedantin. I am not at all a dry-lip Vedantin. I am a practical Vedantin.

I practise and advocate the Yoga of Synthesis. I practise Ahimsa [non-violence], Satyam [purity] and Brahmacharya [celibacy].

Renunciation of egoism alone constitutes the renunciation of all. Doership or enjoyership arises through the idea of 'I'.

The word Guru contains two letters—*Gu* and *Ru*. Gu means darkness and Ru means the dispeller. Being the dispeller of the darkness of ignorance, the teacher is called Guru.

GURU AND DIKSHA (INITIATION)

Yoga should be learnt from a Guru. It is he who will recognise the class to which the aspirant belongs and prescribe suitable Sadhana. The reason for the early downfall of the majority of aspirants is that they imagine themselves to be qualified to adopt the highest form of Yoga at the beginning. The qualified aspirant will be humble enough to approach a Guru, surrender himself to the Guru and serve and learn from him.

Diksha is the giving of the Mantra by the Guru. Initiation gives spiritual knowledge and destroys sin. As one lamp is lit at the flame of another, so the divine Sakti within Mantra is communicated from Guru to the disciple.

Initiation tears the veil of mystery and enables the disciple to grasp the hidden truth behind scriptural texts. The Guru only, by Diksha, will give the right perspective in which to study the scriptures. He will flash his torch of Self-Realisation on the truth within them.

SIDDHI

Siddhi is perfection. A Siddha is one who has attained perfection or Self-realisation through Sadhana. Literally Siddhi means success, achievement, attainment and fruition of all kinds.

One may attain Siddhi in speech, Mantra, Yoga, etc. The greatest of all Siddhis is liberation or Moksha, freedom from the cycle of births and deaths, and union with Para Brahma or the Supreme Being.

The aspirant should not pursue siddhis, as he may misuse the powers. He should ignore them as they are obstacles in the spiritual path.

I AM PAIN: THY TEACHER

Again and again, it is the search for relief from pain that brings people to the spiritual path. Pain is our teacher, as Swami Sivananda so eloquently says in this poem.

O Man! You curse me, blame me,
You hate me and frown on me,
You think I am cruel and heartless;
You try to slay me with anaesthetics,
With Chloroform and Bromides;
You attack me with anodynes,
Sedatives and opiates;
You phone to the doctors
And run to the hospitals,
You fly to Vienna and the hill stations,
You wire to your friends and relations;
You approach the saints of Himalayas
For Buties or herbs;
You do Mrityunjaya Japa and Havan,
You burn incense and pray—
To kill the Teacher Who warns you,
Who comes to help and bless you!

II

I am not your enemy—
I am your sincere friend!
I am a messenger from God,
I am an Angel from heaven—
To teach you wisdom,
To instill in your heart
Mercy and dispassion,
To turn your mind towards God,
To destroy your intense clinging
To things mundane—
That are perishable and illusory.
I am your guide and silent Teacher!
I am pain, the best thing in this world!
I am an eye-opener, soul-awakener,
I am an inspirer and thriller;
I came to remind you of God,
To point to you the Divine Path,
To make you desist from evil ways,
To make you practise virtues, good habits.
You have really misunderstood me.
I am a mental Vritti in the mind-lake,
I am only absence of pleasure,
I co-exist with pleasure—
I am the other side of the coin of pleasure-pain.
I am the cause of the starting of philosophy,
I am the cause for man's Purushartha—
I am the cause for man's aspiration:
I set the mind of philosophers to think,
I make the Yogis to start Sadhana,
I make the sages to practise meditation,
I make a worldly man a Super man.

III

You failed to observe the laws of health—
The rules of hygiene and right-living,
You took Rajasic and Tamasic foods,
You were not regular in doing exercise,
You did not practise Pranayama and Asanas,
You did not pray and meditate;
You were immoderate in your food—
You did not take a balanced diet,
You did not bask in the sun,
You slept in ill-ventilated rooms.
You took too much of sweetmeats,
You drank impure water,
You hated and injured your neighbours,
You were lustful, malicious and greedy,
You took meat, fish and eggs
And developed gout, rheumatism and albuminaria
You married a third wife,
You were a heavy smoker in the club,
You drank liquors in the hotels;
You took bribes and cheated in business;
You twisted the truth in the courts,
And by clever advocacy
Sent innocent men
To the prison and the gallows.
You injected water into the veins
And charged heavily for injections:—
And so, I come to you
To heal, teach and guide!

IV

Understand now at least
My secret and good nature,
My interest in your well-being.
Lead a virtuous life,
Practise simple living and high thinking,

Lead a natural life,
Observe the laws of health and hygiene—
Eat simple food, a well-balanced diet,
Take only vegetarian diet;
Practise Ahimsa, Satyam, Brahmacharya,
Lead the Life Divine,
Remain as a Brahmacharin,
Or better still, take to Sannyasa
After equipping yourself with 'four'.
Attend the Sadhana Weeks,
Practise Sadhana in Ananda Kutir,
And the Training Courses,
Go through the "Divine Life" magazine,
Study "Spiritual lessons," "Aphorisms,"
"The Necessity for Sannyasa"
And practise the precepts contained therein;
Remember Lord Viswanath always,
Take bath in the Ganges and purify.
Then I will depart and leave you,
I will not trouble you any longer.
Love me, believe me, heed my message
I will give you peace, bliss, immortality,
I will surely bless you:
This is my definite promise, friend!
Good bye, comrade! Be cheerful!

SUGGESTED READING LIST

Mantras Words of Power first appeared in 1980. Literature which has since been published and deemed relevant for those interested in pursuing the study of Mantra is asterisked (*).

*ALPER, HARVEY P. *Mantra.* Albany: State University of New York Press, 1989. A scholarly collection of essays on Mantra in the Kasmiri-Shaivism tradition.

ANDREWS, DONALD HATCH. *The Symphony of Life.* Lees Summit, Montana: Unity Books, 1966. A poetic understanding of the unseen, unheard universe as musical vibration by a renowned chemist.

AUROBINDO GHOSE, SRI. *The Mother.* Pondicherry, India: Sri Aurobindo Ashram, 1928. An illuminating and inspiring celebration of the feminine creative power.

*AVALON, ARTHUR [Sir John Woodroffe]. *Shakti and Shakta.* Madras, India: Ganesh & Co. (Madras) Ltd., 1951. Mantra practice as the direction of power to achieve specific spiritual goals in the tradition of Kundalini Yoga.

*_____.*The Serpent Power.* Madras, India: Ganesh & Co. (Madras) Ltd., 1953. The role of Mantra in the Kundalini system, with reference to traditional texts and commentaries.

*AVALON, ARTHUR & ELLEN. *Hymns to the Goddess.* Madras, India: Ganesh & Co. (Madras) Ltd., 1952. The books by Avalon listed here, together with *The Garland of Letters* (see Woodroffe), refer to the significance of Mantra as described in the classic texts of India.

*_____. *Principles of Tantra*. Ganesh & Co., 1952.

*_____. *The Great Liberation*. Ganesh & Co., 1953.

*_____. *Hymn to Kali Karpuradi-Stotra*. Ganesh & Co., 1953.

*BACOVCIN, HELEN. *The Way of A Pilgrim and the Pilgrim Continues His Way*. New York: Doubleday, 1978. A devotional guide to the use of Mantra from a Christian perspective.

*BERENDT, JOACHIM-ERNST. *The World Is Sound: Nada Brahma*. Rochester, Vermont: Destiny Books, 1991. Insights in how to approach sound for spiritual development; notes and discography.

*_____. *The Third Ear*. New York, New York: Henry Holt Books, 1992. Essays on awareness through listening; notes with discography.

Bhajans at Yasodhara. Spokane, Washington: Timeless Books, 1989. Western musical notation for bhajans or songs popular at Yasodhara Ashram, Swami Radha's Ashram in British Columbia, Canada.

BLOFELD, JOHN. *Mantras: Sacred Words of Power*. New York: E.P. Dutton & Co., 1977. Mantra is described as a vehicle for the discovery of our innate divinity.

*BRIANCHANINOV, BISHOP IGNATIUS. *On The Prayer Of Jesus*. Shaftesbury, Dorset: Element Books, 1987. An early 19th century essay on the use of the Jesus Prayer by a Russian Orthodox Bishop.

EASWARAN, EKNATH. *The Unstruck Bell*. Berkeley, California: Nilgiri Press, 1993. A well-known popular introduction to Mantra, previously titled *The Mantram Handbook*.

*FEUERSTEIN, GEORG. *Sacred Paths*. Paul Brunton Philosophic Foundation, 1991. Readable, insightful introductions conveying the spirit of Yoga.
*_____. *The Philosophy of Classical Yoga*. New York: St. Martin's Press, 1980.

_____. The Essence of Yoga. New York: Grove Press, 1976.

GOVINDA, LAMA ANAGARIKA. *Creative Meditation and Multi-Dimensional Consciousness.* Wheaton, Illinois: Quest Books, 1974. The use of Mantra in the Tibetan Vajrayana tradition.

HAMEL, PETER MICHAEL. *Through Music to the Self.* Boulder, Colorado: Shambhala, 1979. A cross-cultural investigation of sound and its principles, methods, and exercises for experimentation with the power of sound.

*HOFFSTEIN, ROBERT M. *The English Alphabet.* New York: Kaedmon Publishing Co., 1975. The relationship between sound and meaning is described in terms of the mystical aspects of English letters and words.

KHAN, HAZRAT INYAT. *The Mysticism of Sound: the power of the word; cosmic language.* vol.2. Geneva, Switzerland: Servire Wassenaar, 1962.

*KHAN, SUFI (HAZRAT) INAYAT. *Music.* Geneva, Switzerland: Sufi Publishing Company, 1988.

LALITA. *Choose Your Own Mantra.* New York: Bantam, 1978.

*MAIN, JOHN. *Word Into Silence.* Ramsey, New Jersey: Paulist Press, 1981. A Christian approach to the use of Mantra in meditation.

Mantras, Bhajans, Songs at Yasodhara Ashram. Kootenay Bay, British Columbia: Yasodhara Ashram Society, 1979. Western musical notation for the music used at Yasodhara Ashram.

*MUKHYANANDA, SWAMI. *Om, Gayatri and Sadhya.* Mylapore, Madras: Sri Ramakrishna Math, 1989. A brief introduction to the Gayatri Mantra, the major Vedic Mantra.

The Musical Scale and the Scheme of Evolution. Mt. Ecclesia, Oceanside, California: The Rosicrucian Fellowship, 1949.

*NIERENBERG, GERARD I. and CALERO, HENRY. *Meta-Talk.* New York: Trident Press, 1973. Sensitivity to the hidden meanings in speech is stimulated by this book.

RADHA, SWAMI SIVANANDA. *Kundalini: Yoga For The West.* Spokane, Washington: Timeless Books, 1993. This classic text on Kundalini Yoga for the western reader presents practical methods to build a firm foundation for spiritual development and explains the use of Mantra practice in this context.

_____. *Mantras, Songs of Yoga.* Spokane, Washington: Timeless Books, 1973. A variety of Mantras chanted by Swami Radha. Sound cassette or record.

_____. *Power of Mantras.* Spokane, Washington: Timeless Books, 1974. Swami Radha provides a guide to establishing a Mantra practice and explains several Mantras. Sound cassette.

*_____. *Ave Maria: Most Beautiful Mother.* Spokane, Washington: Timeless Books, 1993. A Christian prayer to Mary presented for use in a way similar to a Mantra. Sound cassette.

*_____. *Radhe Govinda.* Spokane, Washington: Timeless Books, 1993. A Mantra depicting the love of the soul in pursuit of the Divine. Sound cassette.

*_____. Sri *Rama.* Spokane, Washington: Timeless Books, 1993. A Mantra invoking the power to overcome ignorance and self-will for the victory of the spirit. Sound cassette.

*_____. *Hari Om.* Spokane, Washington: Timeless Books, 1975. A Mantra calling upon the healing forces to preserve the body and mind for the purpose of attaining Self-Realization. Sound cassette.

*_____. Om N*ama Sivaya.* Spokane, Washington: Timeless Books, 1976. A Mantra calling upon the Divine to overcome the obstacles of illusion. Sound cassette.

*_____. *Om Krishna Guru.* Spokane, Washington: Timeless Books, 1990. A Mantra which calls to the Guru within and to the human Guru who guides the individual. Sound cassette.

*_____. *Om Tara Tuttare.* Spokane, Washington: Timeless Books, 1989. An invocation of the Buddhist Goddess of Compassion. Sound cassette.

RAMDAS, SWAMI. *In Quest of God.* Bombay: Bharatiya Vidya Bhavan, 1961. An inspiring story illustrating devotion to Mantra by a master with whom Swami Radha lived and studied in India.

*RUDHYAR, DANE. *The Rebirth of Hindu Music.* New York: Samuel Weiser, 1979. A dated, yet enlivened monograph on the living nature of sound.

*_____. *The Magic of Tone and the Art of Music.* Boulder, Colorado: Shambhala, 1982. A challenge to consider the meaning of sound and its role in the transformation of consciousness.

SIVANANDA SARASWATI, SWAMI. *Concentration and Meditation.* Himalayas, India: The Divine Life Society, 1975.

_____. *Japa Yoga: a comprehensive treatise of Mantra-Shastra.* Himalayas, India: The Divine Life Society, 1972.

_____. *Music as Yoga.* Rishikesh, India: The Yoga-Vedanta Forest University, 1956.

_____. *Tantra Yoga, Nada Yoga, and Kriya Yoga.* Rishikesh, India: Yoga-Vedanta Forest Academy, 1955. Concise information on the essentials of Mantra in the traditional context of Tantra Yoga.

*TAIMNI, I.K. *Gayatri.* Adyar, Madras: Theosophical Publishing House, 1989. An outline of the use of the Gayatri Mantra in the context of worship and meditation.

*TOMATIS, ALFRED A. *The Conscious Ear: My Life of Transformation Through Listening.* Translated by Stephen Lushington and Billie M. Thompson. Barrytown, New York: Station Hill Press, 1992. Listening as a therapeutic vehicle.

TYBERG, JUDITH M. *The Language of the Gods.* Los Angeles: East-West Cultural Center, 1974.

WHORF, BENJAMIN LEE. *Language, Thought and Reality,* selected writings. Edited by John B. Carroll. Cambridge, Mass: M.I.T. Press, 1956.

*WILLIS, JANICE DEAN. *The Diamond Light.* New York: Simon and Shuster, 1973. A clear, detailed introduction to Mantra in Tibetan Buddhist meditation practice.

*WINSTON, SHIRLEY RABB. *Music as the Bridge.* Virginia Beach, Virginia: A.R.E. Press, 1972. A review of the readings of Edgar Cayce on music and sound in relation to spiritual development.

*WOODROFFE, SIR JOHN [Arthur Avalon, pseud.]. *Garland of Letters.* Madras, India: Ganesh & Co., (Madras) Ltd., 1922.

*YOGANANDA, PARAMAHANSA. *Cosmic Chants.* Los Angeles: Self-Realisation Fellowship, 1991. A charming collection of devotional songs, with western musical notation, accessible to the western ear.

*YOGI HARI. *Bhajan, Kirtan, Slokas and Chants.* Fort Lauderdale, Florida: Nada Productions, 1991. An introduction to traditional Hindustani devotional music, with Indian musical notation, companion to a set of audio tapes.

ZUCHERKANDL, VICTOR. *Sound and Symbol: music and the external world.* Translated from the German by W.R. Trask. Bollingen Series XLIV. Princeton, New Jersey: Princeton University Press, 1956.

INDEX

acceptance 40
Adonai 78
Adwaita 138, 148
affirmations 89
Aham Brahmasmi 94
ahimsa 143, 154, 158
ambition 117
Ananda Lahari 84
anger 52, 126, 133, 138
Aristotle xxvii
asana 19, 53, 54, 120, 157
aspirant
  advanced, as teacher 143
  and prayer 1
  faith of 139
  maturing of 65
  qualifications of 103,
    107, 139, 140, 142, 143,
    145, 147, 153, 154
Atman 149
attachment 50, 80, 88
AUM 45, 66, 68, 77
  how to chant 66
  meditation on 67
Ave Maria 31, 76
awareness 41, 44, 50, 57,
  59, 97

Badrinath 151
bhakti 153

Bhakti Yoga xxvi, 9, 29, 42
Bible 82, 89
biblical phrases, chanting 89
bija 2, 4, 5
bliss 41
body 17
body-mind 42
Brahma Vidya 151
Brahmacharya 143, 158
brahmacharya 109, 154,
  158
Brahman 66, 94, 139,
  145, 149, 155
breath 22, 33, 38, 39,
  51, 52, 53, 78, 79, 87,
  88, 124
breathing techniques 23
Buddha 31, 72, 78, 142
Buddhism xix
  Tibetan 10, 72, 114

cancer 119
celibacy 143, 153
chakras xxvi
chanting 21, 39
  at temple doors 137
  biblical phrases 89
  effects of 10
  extended periods 22, 57,
    118, 121

for friends 56
for healing, how to 95
Guru's name 78
individual matter 49
length of 49
Lord's name 137
Lord's Prayer 89
mechanical 86
sound of 51
speed of 51
teacher's name 54
variations 51, 78
with concentration 56
Christ 30, 31
Christ Consciousness 90
Christianity 4
commitment
disciple to Guru 105
Guru to disciple 102
initiation and 108
ritual and 125
to Mantra 104
written 18
compassion 96, 97
development of 97
healing and 97
Mother of 75
Siva and 80
competition xxi
concentration 37, 42, 45,
51, 53, 56, 57, 58, 78,
79, 93, 124, 136

Confucius xxviii
consciousness 2, 5, 11, 39,
68, 81, 149
Cosmic Consciousness 6,
132, 152
Cosmic Lover 68
criticalness 131
cross 58, 70, 116

cults 138
Dalai Lama 114
death 135
dehypnotizing 44
depression xx
desire, imagination and 30
desires xxvi, 32
despair 39
Devata 2, 3, 4, 6, 29, 32
defined 3
devotion 9, 29, 56, 76,
89, 103, 136, 143,
147, 154
as emotions transformed
117
between student and
teacher 139
chanting with 10
in healing 95
in women 43
mala and 17
Mantra as 37
symbol of 32
to Guru 136, 140, 150,
152
diary 22, 50, 86
diksha 104, 146, 154
disciple (see also aspirant)
5, 11, 102, 103, 107,
138
relationship with Guru
2, 11, 43, 102, 104, 105,
107, 140, 141, 143,
146, 150
discipline 50

discrimination 42, 50,
52, 144
Divine Energy 4, 40
Divine Light 67, 88

Divine Light Invocation
 85, 88
Divine Light Invocation
 Mantra 88
Divine Mother xvi, xix,
 5, 16, 22, 31, 72, 76,
 78, 84, 85, 86, 114
 Mary xix
 Mother of Compassion
 xix
Divine Mother Mantra 85
Divine, the
 images of 63
 in everyone 45, 88
 manifestation of 23
 personal concept of 4
 personal relationship with
 3, 29, 64, 118
 union with xxv
doubt 23, 52, 78, 136,
 139, 151
dreams 16, 53, 107, 133
duality, male-female xvi
Dvapara Yuga xxvi

ear 30, 45
ego 18, 21, 24, 29, 38,
 42, 43, 55, 59, 66, 80,
 131, 140, 150, 152, 153
 illness and 94
egoism 50, 66, 67, 138, 1
 40, 141, 151, 154
Elohim 78
embroider 32, 113
emotion(s) 17, 22, 38, 40,
 41, 57, 58, 68, 71, 80,
 89, 93, 118, 121, 123,
 124, 126
 as source of strength 40
 breath and 40, 52

channeled to Divine
 40, 54
control of 38, 39
during chanting 52
given back to Divine 40,
 41, 52, 58
indulgence in 23, 40, 52
offered to Divine 38
purification of 39, 50
refined 39, 67
Self-Realization and 44
transformed to devotion
 117
voice and 39
energy 41, 43, 53, 70,
 88, 140
 as creation 5
 as male and female aspects
 of God 5
 divine 4
 released in chanting 5
 Siva as xvi
extrasensory perception 23
eye(s) 20, 22, 30, 45, 75,
 113, 139

fainting 22
faith 136, 140, 143, 153
fear 39, 123, 124, 139
feelings 38, 39, 58, 76
feelings, 89
female principle 76
flowers xvi, 30, 31, 32,
 81, 102, 124, 125
flute 64, 66
food 86, 131, 157
forgiveness 94, 97

generosity 144

God-Realization 17, 20,
64, 141, 152
Goddess of the Spoken Word
5
God's child 41, 52, 75
God's servant 52, 82
Gopala 148
Gospel of St. John 1
gratitude 54, 57, 78, 80,
98, 107, 131
Greeks xxvii
gunas 70
Guru xxi, 2, 5, 11, 16,
43, 54, 56, 70, 78, 101,
108, 120, 135, 136,
138, 154
-shopping 102
characteristics of 138
choosing 140, 152
divine nature of 145
doubts about 102, 108
meaning 154
necessity of 151
parting from 105
photo of 143
pseudo 141
serving 152
true 101
types 146
women and choice of 108
Guru Nanak 138
Guru-disciple relationship
(see also disciple) 11
Gurubhakti 140

habit xix
Hail Mary 76
handmaiden, of Divine
Mother 86
Hari Om 31, 51, 64, 77,

79, 89, 126
chanting other words 78
for chanting Guru's name
78
variations in chanting 78
when to chant 78
harmony xxvii, 2, 10,
66, 137
Hatha Yoga xxvi, 31, 53
healing xxvi, 93, 98
and sound xxvi
Cosmic Light and 98
ego and 94
Hari Om and 77
rejected 98
health 94, 158
heart 63, 66, 69, 119,
122, 147, 150
Higher Self
38, 42, 101, 120
Hinduism 76
humility 42, 43, 52, 55,
80, 94, 95, 103, 107,
124, 132
healing and 94
illness and 94
in women 43
humor 104
hypnotism 43, 44

Icarus xx
ideals 23
ignorance 80, 140
illness 80
advantages 94
ego and 94
necessity of 95
returning 98
illusion 80

image xvi, xxvi, 3, 30,
    53, 57, 81, 124
  as rival of God 64
  of Divine 63, 70
  of Divine Mother 86
  produced by singing xxvii
  use during practice 29
imagination 23, 30, 32
  cultivating 30, 33
immorality xxvi
imperfection 136
initiation 11, 56, 101,
    102, 109, 141, 143,
    146, 154
  brahmacharya 109
  responsibilities of
    102, 104, 108
  sanyasa 109
inspiration
    58, 66, 82, 88, 142
intellect 43, 123, 124, 149
intellectual doubts 52
intellectual pride 124
intellectual, the 42
intuition 132, 139, 149
Iron Age xxvi
Ishta Devata 29, 146
Ishta Mantra 16, 64

Japa
  alternated 57
  Likhita 10, 57, 133
  Manasika 10, 57, 133
  Upamsu 10, 133
  Vaikhari 10, 133
Japa Yoga 9, 16, 42
Jericho xxvii
Jesus 4, 70, 71, 95, 97,
    105, 116
Jnana 138

Jnana Yoga xxvi, 9, 42
joy 39, 41, 52, 66
judgment 20, 97
Kali Yuga xxvi, 12
Kali Yuga Keval Namah
    Adhara, xxvi
karma 96, 97, 105, 106
Karma Yoga 9, 140
kilaka 2, 5, 114
koan 10
Krishna xvi, xix, xxi, 4,
    64, 66, 68, 70, 71, 77,
    95, 115, 144, 150
  as image for chanting 30
  as lover 64
  symbolism 70
Krishna Invocation 68, 69
Kudu-Kudu 136
Kundalini 139
  system xxvi
Kundalini Yoga 31

Lakshmi 78
language xxvii, 10
liberation 43, 132, 155
Light 23, 32, 33, 88,
    95, 149
Likhita Japa 10, 57, 133
loneliness 39
Lord's Prayer 89, 90
lotus 58, 67, 70, 107
  posture 19
  visualization 23
love xxvii, 9, 29, 30, 39,
    40, 42, 52, 53, 54,
    56, 64, 71, 76, 104,
    141, 147, 149
  affair with God 49
  self-love 40
lower self 42

mala xix, 16, 17, 18, 115
Manasika Japa 10, 57, 133
mandala 10
Mantra
  alternating practices 10
  as blessing 11
  as devotion 37
  as shield 39
  at work 58
  changing 16, 65, 154
  chanting several 16, 65
  choosing 16, 65, 141,
    153
  concentration and 37
  continuously in mind 38
  control of breath and 38
  control of emotions and
    38
  creation of xxvi
  defined 1, 2, 12
  deity of 63
  Devatas in 3, 4
  Divine Mother
    85, 87, 125
  divined by rishis xxvi
  dreams and 53
  energy of 2, 43
  fear and 38
  for each person 16, 64
  for material benefits 84
  given by parents 106
  goal of 6
  Hatha Yoga and 53
  healing and 77, 93, 98
  household tasks and
    53, 133
  hypnotism and 43
  imperfection and 136
  intellectual explanation of
    2, 64

  linking Guru and disciple
    102
  listening to 11
  meaning of words 64
  mental repetition 10
  of Divine Light Invocation
    85, 88
  of the heart 63
  power of xv, 2, 4, 11,
    12, 22
  power of, control of 23
  power of, self-generating
    5, 11
  power of, superceding
    words 11
  pronunciation of 56
  purification and 37, 38
  received from Guru 11
  received in dream 107
  recited aloud 58
  recited without raga 84
  refinement of senses and
    45
  rishis and 2
  self-generating power of
    4, 5, 104, 121
  silent 57
  six aspects of 2
  sleep and 43, 133
  sound and image 3
  source of 1
  spoken aloud 10
  surrender to 43
  tape 55, 65, 133
  to counteract negative
    words 96
  to counteract prejudice 44
  transmission of 2
  whispered 10
  work and 132
  written 10, 57

Mantra practice 29
  breathing 20
  changes to 59
  critical points in 50
  excuses to stop 15
  extended
    57, 85, 89, 118, 121
  how to 21, 30
  ideals and 15
  length of 10, 18, 49,
    55, 119, 124, 126
  mental impasse in xv,
    xix
  place 19
  posture 19
  reflection and 50
  setting up 18
  spiritual diary and 50
  time 18
  walking xx
Mantra Shastra 12
Mantra Yoga xxvi, xxviii,
  3, 6, 9, 38, 42, 59
  defined 9
mantric power 56
marriage xx, 105
  spiritual 102
Mary xix, 4
maya xxvi, 6
mayurasana 54
meditation xv, xvi, xxvi,
  10, 11, 66, 137, 150,
  154, 156
melody xxvii, xxviii, 2,
  10, 21, 56, 76, 139
memory 51, 124
mental background noises
  41, 51
mercy 29
Milarepa 142

mind 43, 50, 69, 87,
  136, 138, 145
  as deceiver 114, 151
  as elephant 51
  as laboratory 49
  body and 42
  carnal 55
  clearing 19
  creations of 70
  creativity of 63, 64
  discrimination and 42
  effect of chanting on 10
  emotions and 123
  focusing xvi, 10, 17,
    22, 29, 31, 44, 51,
    58, 89
  healing of 95
  illuminated by AUM 66
  images and 30, 33
  impasses 50
  intellectual 43
  irrational 123
  limited 4, 63, 93
  manifestations of
    xx, 23, 44
  memory and 51
  monkey- 88, 124
  observation of 15
  pain and 95
  polarity of 94
  purification of
    18, 38, 67, 132
  rational 119, 122
  reasoning 59
  relaxed 93
  resistance of xv, xix,
    xxi, 10, 30, 57, 85, 98
  restlessness of
    17, 30, 50, 65, 78, 133
  stillness of 41

surrender of 29, 59
vibrations of 32
Moksha 148, 151, 155
moods 41
Mount Kailas 81
Mount Meru 17, 18
mudra 85
music xxvii
   arithmetic and xxvii
   Indian 3
   lawlessness and xxviii
   of the spheres xxvii, 45
   rock xxvii

Nada Brahmananda 56
Nada Yoga xxv, xxviii, 16
negativity 118
Neti-Neti Doctrine 141

obstacles 50, 64, 80, 123
Om (see also AUM)
   5, 66, 78
Om Krishna Guru 70
Om Namah Sivaya 54, 64,
   80, 81, 96, 112,
   113, 120
Om Sri Rama Jaya Rama 81
Om Tara 31, 72, 75, 113
Ouspensky xxvii
out-of-body experience xxi
over-sensitivity 39

padmasana 19
pain 95, 105, 155
pairs of opposites 87
Parable of the Sower 105
Parma Akasha 1
past lives 38
Patanjali 149

peace 69
peacock pose 54
pearl 80, 133
personality aspects 42
pets 88
pillar (see also kilaka) 2
pleasure 85, 86, 156
power(s)
   generative, of Mantra 43
   manifest xvi
   of siddhis 23
   of silence 87
   of sound xxvi
   of words 3
   unmanifest xvi, xx
   yogic 105, 131, 136
prana 19, 53
Pranava 66
pranayama 157
prayer 1, 20, 22, 30, 32,
   58, 76, 86, 89, 93, 95
pride 52, 123, 138,
   140, 141
   of intellect 124
primal sound 3, 5
prostration 43, 85
protection 31, 124
psychic 112
psychology 65
purification 37, 43, 50,
   53, 94, 133, 140
Purushotthamananda 104
Pythagorus xxvii

Radha 71, 78, 114, 124
Radhe Govinda 71, 72
raga xxvii, 2, 10, 55
   correct use of 10, 56
   defined 2
   key of 3

Raja Yoga 9
Rama 81, 82, 144
Ramakrishna 107
Ramdas 82, 106
reflection 50, 86, 89
    in Hatha Yoga 54
reincarnation 38, 43, 44,
    106, 151
    knowledge reappearing in
    131
    of Guru and disciples 107
relaxation 93
renunciation 154
repetitions xx, 50, 76
    counting xix, 16
    in one breath 51
    number of 55
    variations 52
resentment 118
rhythm xxvii
rishis xxvi, 1, 2, 21, 31
ritual 31, 32, 124

sacrifice xxvi, 153
sadhana 66, 150, 151,
    154, 155, 156, 158
Sakta 31
Sakti xvi, 2, 5, 104, 154
sakti 141
samsara 2
Sankara 84, 144, 154
Sanskrit 56, 77
sanyas 106, 109, 158
sanyasin 106, 108, 143,
    152, 153
Saraswati 78
satsang 111, 147
Satya Yuga xxv
satyam 154, 158
seed sound (see also bija) 2

self
    -analysis 144
    -centeredness 71, 80
    -denial 144
    -development 133
    -glorification 43
    -gratification 43
    -importance 43, 66
    -justification 43
    -love 40
    -pity 52
    -restraint 144
    -surrender 152
    -will 42, 43, 66
Self-Realization 11, 12,
    39, 44, 45, 63, 102,
    140, 154
selfishness 43, 95
selfless service 98, 140, 144
sensation 23
senses 45, 90, 131
sexuality 108
Shabda 3, 5
Shakespeare 112
shawl 19, 21
siddha 155
siddhasana 19
siddhi 155
siddhis 23
silence 125
sin 104, 154
sincerity 103, 104
single-pointedness 10, 15,
    29, 42, 50, 51, 52, 56,
    63, 78, 89, 90, 93
    and distress 41
sinner 94, 97, 98
Siva xvi, 4, 16, 31, 64,
    80, 81, 95
    as destroyer of obstacles
    31, 80

Lord of Hatha Yoga 31
Lord of Kundalini 31
Siva stone 31
Sivananda xv, xvi, xx,
    xxi, xxvi, 3, 22, 56, 66,
    103, 104, 106, 107,
    108
sleep 43, 133
snakes 54, 85
soul 69, 71, 98
sound xxvi, 53, 64, 87,
    119, 120, 124
  as union of breath and
    intellect 10
  effects on hearer xxvii
  essence of 3
  image and xxvi
  power to influence human
    thought xxvii
  primal 1
  production of 51
speech 144
spine 19
spiritual baby 41, 49, 153
spiritual dryness 105
spiritual experience 6
spiritual movies xxi
spiritualists 112
star 75
stillness 41, 69, 81
subconscious 43
Subramanya 54
sukhasana 19
surrender 29, 43, 58, 66,
    68, 94, 96, 141
  healing and 97
symbol xvi, 32
  blue xxi

tape 41, 55, 65, 133

Tara 72, 95, 113, 114, 125
  Green 75
  Red 113
  White 72
tears 52
television 44, 55, 96
temptation 23, 30
time 75
toys 50
Treta Yuga xxvi
truth 44
two worlds 23

unity 12
Upamsu Japa 10
Upanishads 1, 150

Vach 1, 3
Vaikhari Japa 10, 133
vairagya 144, 145
vanity 54
Vedanta 109
Vedas 138, 144
vibration xxvi, 3, 16, 22,
    32, 64, 97, 120, 138
  form and 3
  living center of 2
  Mantra focusing 1
virasana 19
Virgin Mother 31
Vishnu 31, 77
viveka 144
voice xx, 45, 52, 53,
    56, 78, 117, 124
  adjusting to Mantra 21
  emotions and 39, 40
  taped 57
  volume of 51
vritti 156

walking, as spiritual practice
xx
water 31, 32, 70, 125, 157
will-power
5, 50, 52, 55, 126
willingness 124, 125
wisdom
9, 29, 32, 154, 156
women 43, 108
worship xxvi, 29, 32,
33, 85, 86, 149
chanting and xvi, 30
images and 30
of Divine Mother 76, 114
of Guru 142, 143, 146,
152
of Siva 31
of the Divine 3, 32, 152
ritual for xvi, 30, 124
work as 140

Yoga
Mantra 59
yoga 132, 151
Bhakti xxvi, 9, 29, 42
goal of xxv
Hatha xxvi, 31, 53
Japa 9, 16, 42
Jnana xxvi, 9, 42
Karma 9, 140
Kundalini xxvi, 31
Mantra xxvi, xxviii,
6, 9, 38, 42
Nada xxviii, 16
of action 9
of knowledge and wisdom
9, 42
of love and devotion
9, 29, 42
of selfless service 9

of sound xxv, xxviii, 16
paths of xxv, xxviii, 9
practice of several
recommended 9
Yoga Sutras of Patanjali 9
yuga xxv
Dvapara xxvi
Kali xxvi, 12
Satya xxv
Treta xxvi

Zen 10

About the Author

For more than 35 years Swami Sivananda Radha has expressed the most profound teachings of the East in simple, clear and straightforward language, making them more accessible to those who wish to attain to Higher Consciousness. Author of many classic books on Eastern philosophy, she has, through her experience with yoga, gained a true understanding of Eastern symbolism and an ability to communicate this knowledge to the Western seeker.

She has lectured all over North America and internationally at universities, colleges, churches, and psychological institutes, and is one of the most widely-known spiritual teachers today. Translations of her books are available in many languages, including French, Spanish, Italian, German, and Dutch.

Classes and Workshops

Workshops and classes based on Swami Radha's teachings are available from her Ashram in Canada—Yasodhara Ashram—and at affiliated centers, called Radha Houses, located in urban communities internationally.

For further information on programs offered by Yasodhara Ashram or the Radha Houses (including a vacation and yoga retreat center in Merida, Mexico) write: The Program Secretary, Yasodhara Ashram, Box 9MP, Kootenay Bay, B.C., Canada VOB 1X0.

Further Inquiries

To obtain a free catalogue of all books, audio tapes, and video tapes by Swami Sivananda Radha please write: Timeless Books, PO Box 3543MP, Spokane, WA 99220-3543.

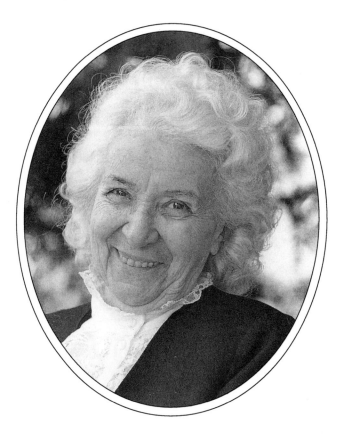